Henri Chenot

PURE HEALTH

The secrets of well-being and harmony

In collaboration with Jean-Luc Suchet

JOHN BLAKE

Published by Metro Publishing
an imprint of John Blake Publishing Ltd
3 Bramber Court, 2 Bramber Road,
London W14 9PB, England

www.johnblakepublishing.co.uk

www.facebook.com/Johnblakepub facebook
twitter.com/johnblakepub twitter

First published in paperback in 2011
Previously published as *Cure de Santé*

ISBN: 978 1 84358 368 4

British Library Cataloguing-in-Publication Data:

A catalogue record for this book is available from the British Library.

Design by www.envydesign.co.uk

Printed in Great Britain by CPI Mackays, Chatham, ME5 8TD

3 5 7 9 10 8 6 4 2

Papers used by John Blake Publishing are natural, recyclable products
made from wood grown in sustainable forests. The manufacturing processes
conform to the environmental regulations of the country of origin.

CONTENTS

FOREWORD

It's better to look after your health
than to cure illness

After 40 years of experience and welcoming thousands of patients to my detox centre, I have decided to write this book to share my thoughts and knowledge on the subject of detox, vitality and achieving harmony through your weight. My way of working is to keep things constantly updated and refreshed according to new scientific developments.

This scientific supervision is carried out by the Academy of Biontology which I set up in the spa town of Merano, northern Italy. But what is biontology? It is the study of the essence of life and its evolution – 'bio' meaning 'life', and 'ontology' referring to the area of metaphysics that deals with the nature of being.

Everyone deserves to benefit from the results of our experiments. Over the years, my colleagues and I have given thousands of lectures, and at Merano we suggest many sources of information to our patients – I firmly believe that people who come to the academy shouldn't just be content to go through a treatment, they should understand it in depth in order to gain the best results.

The right to know is of prime importance, as it's the only way in which we can respect our freedom as individuals. Once we fully appreciate each situation, we can take responsibility and make informed choices and reasoned decisions, which is vital when undertaking any changes related to our health. I've seen too many patients believing any old theory and acting in any old way and putting themselves in danger through sheer ignorance. Today, in developed countries, our methods of communication and teaching are ever more effective, and everyone should have access to this knowledge. Teaching people about health should start as early as primary school.

Of course, knowing about something doesn't necessarily mean knowing *how* to do it. This calls for even more in-depth knowledge. Unfortunately, too often this know-how comes in the form of ready-made, impersonal and generalised approaches which pop up time and again in the new-year and spring issues of magazines. It's as if there are as many diets as there are high-street fashions, and you can change them according to how you feel on a daily basis, but lots of these diets can represent real dangers to our health. Dietetics on the other hand is not a passing trend; it's a serious science that progresses and evolves.

This book aims to increase our knowledge and understanding of ourselves.

CHAPTER ONE

EVERYONE ON
THE SAME MODEL

When we are born, we inherit an extremely impressive 'human machine' equipped with many regular functions that work like clockwork. To live as long as possible in optimum physical condition is an aspiration we can realise by respecting the demands of our machine.

The 'terms and conditions' of the contract with which we have bound our bodies usually guarantee some decades of loyal and untroubled service. All human beings are subject to the same rules, because we are all made according to the same model. However, note that the contract includes particular clauses that take into account the characteristics of each person and call upon us to improve the quality and duration of our lives by making the most of our individual abilities.

It goes without saying that we must be aware of the aforementioned terms and conditions of the contract, in order to know the intrinsic needs of the body, to aim to use it in the best possible way and ensure that this precious vehicle, in which we experience life from birth to death, is working properly.

Its operations are complex, its parts – cells, organs, hormones, fluids – extremely sophisticated. Without food, the body's motor will cease to function. Without its immune system to combat external aggressions, life will remain precarious. And lastly, the body's ageing process is progressive and unavoidable: the operations of the 'body machine' dwindle bit by bit until they cease to function and end up – although hopefully as late as possible – on the scrap heap. This is the law of all our sexual lives, for example, no matter how much we wish it weren't.

Cells – Our Bodies' Building Blocks

The key players in and operators of life – the brain, hormones, organs, bones, muscles, tissues, such as the skin, and fluids – are made up of billions of cells, the building blocks of the human body. Each one contains our DNA, the unique genetic code that forms our identity, and each cell is devoted to a specific function, for example, hepatic cells are chemically the most complex; pancreatic cells are among the most sophisticated because they create enzymes; renal cells, for immunity and elimination, are also incredibly sophisticated. Cells differ according to their function, but also their longevity, for example, the lifespan of intestinal cells is a mere 48 hours, while others renew themselves every seven years.

The brain transmits its orders to a protein in the cell membrane; only this protein is capable of receiving this message and passing it on to the cell. On this signal, nourishing fluid crosses the cell membrane and is transported to the nucleus to provide nourishment. This peripheral protein, along with the protein within cells, disappears every 14 days, so regular renewal of these protein resources is a fundamental necessity in life. The stakes are high because proteins are the body's liquid assets.

Thanks to continuous research, the body continues to open up its secrets and its complexities to us.

Mesenchymal Fluid, Our Driver

Nourishing or mesenchymal fluid is the aqueous

material within which cells bathe. It is made up of fluids – around 16 to 18 litres – but also collagen and elastin fibres, as well as other distinctive substances that ensure a biochemical, metabolic and neuroendocrinal equilibrium of cells.

Across this buffer fluid the cells need to get hold of the nutrients released by the blood capillaries. To allow the nutrients to penetrate, the cells must adjust their polarity so that their membrane becomes permeable. This is how they give the signal of satiety to the brain, through a set of electric charges. Once this work is complete, the cells will modify their polarity again to cause the opposite function.

The Organs, the Mechanics of Our Engine

The appearance of our 'bodywork' – i.e. our skin, or epithelial tissue (superficial epidermis, dermis and hypodermis) – can often reveal what's going on inside. It serves as both a link with, and a visible and palpable barrier to, the outside world. Under the skin is hidden a pool of fats that is in a more or less rounded form. An excess of the fat supply is often attributed to a poor diet.

Each of our organs plays a specific role which only makes sense within the 'network' of the human body.

No organ can survive on its own, and they enjoy good relations among one another. They consist of different types of tissues that are made up of billions of cells that must all continuously regenerate. To help these mechanisms respond on demand, the body requires its energy: food, water, oxygen, etc.

All organs are subject to the same nutritional protocol. If they're provided with their daily ration, they will carry out their roles efficiently: the nervous system maintains communication through and with the senses; the circulation transports nutrients, oxygen and hormones towards the cells; the cardiorespiratory system exchanges gases between the body and the outside air; the digestive system transforms food into nutrients; the urinary and the intestinal systems eliminate waste; the immune system – our 'bodyguard' – defends the body against outside attack; the endocrinal system is the main regulator; and the reproductive system accomplishes the ultimate task of perpetuating the species.

Hormones – Our Switches

To keep the machine running, we're equipped with chemical messengers that operate away from their sites of production in the endocrinal glands.

Hormones are our 'switches': as soon as the brain gives an order, the hormones get busy and allow all the vital processes to take place inside our bodies. In women, a switch is turned on at puberty, another at the start of the menstrual cycle, another during pregnancy. At menopause, the switch turns down the intensity due to a shortage of hormones.

Primary molecules, precursors to hormones called eicosanoids, draw on the nutrients in food: they are partial to fatty acids. Without a fatty acid source, we wouldn't be protected from fluctuations of and disruptions to hormonal levels, as is the case with anorexia: the absence of periods is due to a hormonal imbalance, because the body isn't producing enough oestrogen and progesterone. There are also psychological disorders that bring about a lack of adrenalin.

When they are well fed, eicosanoids differentiate themselves and mutate into hormones. Transported by the blood, the hormones fix themselves on to their specific receptors in order to respond, with unparalleled precision, to all sorts of stimulations. Hormones aren't exclusively linked to sexuality or procreation, of course; besides oestrogen and progesterone in women and testosterone in men, the hormones for the thyroid are very important for circulation levels, immunology and the heart; the ones for the pituitary gland aim to help growth and harmony within the body; those for the pancreas aim to release insulin; and those for the suprarenal gland create adrenalin and corticoids. An excessive or limited production of hormones produces a characteristic disease for each hormone.

The Brain – Our Pilot

Why do we eat? The answer is simple: because our brains tell us to. It's an order. This major organ has important and inescapable duties. One of its priorities is to feed itself and feed the body in order to manage metabolism, to renew cells and to look after itself. These demands must be immediately satisfied.

As the keyholders to the development of our lives and the regeneration of our bodies, each day our brains must obtain a quantity of indispensable material to make the whole body function properly.

What do we understand by the word 'regeneration'? Each day we lose billions of cells, and it is essential that they are reproduced. Equally, we must also produce all the necessary hormones, enzymes and the energy to keep the body temperature at 37°C. If all these conditions aren't met, the body cannot function. Thanks to a complex and fundamental process, it develops a phenomenal amount of nutrients that are intended for all kinds of chemical transformations.

When the body demands its fuel, we experience a rational and legitimate irresistible feeling of hunger. In this book, we will see when and how to curb this demand. One thing's for sure, it's definitely the brain that imposes these desires to satisfy ourselves, and which conveys the body's fundamental needs through a feeling of hunger.

Unfortunately, when an appealing piece of food – such as something sweet and tempting – is near, the pleasures of the eyes can divert the brain's orders. Likewise, a depressive or euphoric state can both lead to an irrational order. We therefore mix up the brain's natural signals with the desire to make up for these psychosomatic shortages or deficiencies with food or drink.

The need to eat can produce unjustified cravings grounded in emotional sensations, irrespective of other factors. Fortunately, we can regulate them. The brain is likely to be distracted by a diet that it's not accustomed to, a diet with multiple flavours, different tastes and concoctions that are slyly hidden in tempting ready-made food. These can distract the brain from its nutritional requirements, tempting it into irrationality with flavoursome bait, and thus the brain loses its bearings, which affects its control of appetite.

The brain carries out our machine's operation with an extraordinary dedication. Because it understands and dictates our need for nutrition to function properly, it deserves the utmost attention.

Chronobiology – Our Cruising Speed

It's not enough to know how to put the right proportion of indispensably healthy food on our plates. We also need to give our bodies what they want when they want, because they are ruled according to a precise regularity.

It is vital to understand that we're subject to inescapable natural daily cycles which require us to renew our food supply every 24 hours. Remember, our bodies can only nourish themselves over this timeframe – before and after aren't the right time.

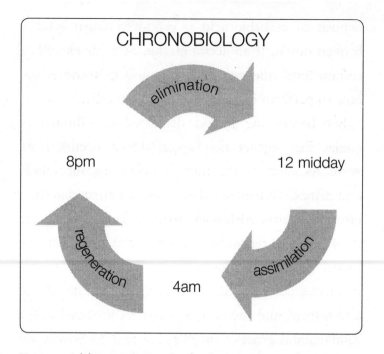

CHRONOBIOLOGY

elimination

8pm

12 midday

regeneration

assimilation

4am

From midday to 8pm, the body is at its peak capacity to eat and digest food; it's the best time to eat and the ideal time to assimilate food, thanks to the lively activity of the digestive system, the liver and the kidneys. Lunchtime and dinnertime fall during this period, and the slow job of breaking down food and rebuilding nutritious substances is set to work. Don't forget, this range of food isn't available to us without first being broken down. This breaking down produces waste, which is why this phase of elimination is so crucial. Depending on the quantity and quality of nutrients we obtain from our diet, a deposit of ascorbic acid is produced when food is broken down. If an accumulation of acids exceeds a certain level, the mesenchymal fluid gels and is not able to perform its job, i.e. to feed the cells.

But before the period dedicated to elimination comes the regeneration stage, which occurs from 8pm. As soon as the flux of nutritious substances diminishes, and their absorption and their digestion are ensured, the metabolic process changes to devote itself to cell regeneration, until around 4 in the morning. Regeneration is most active during this nighttime period when the body is in a state of rest and fasting, and the nutrients can get involved in the fundamental process of cell renewal. This is why we see a drop in body temperature, from 37∞C to 36∞C.

What are the instructions during this period of cell renewal? Don't eat, sleep! After this time, the body will focus its attention on elimination, which lasts for eight hours, from 4am to midday: its priority becomes to free itself from toxic residues.

To assist the elimination and detoxification stage, you should have purifying ingredients such as fruit, natural juices and, above all, water, for breakfast. A large number of Westerners don't observe chronobiology, the precise, fundamental pattern that assists you to respect the three stages.

PURE HEALTH

Another factor that interferes with the assimilation stage is the amount of time given to chewing. You usually start to feel full about a quarter of an hour after you've started eating: so, if you eat fast and don't chew, you will have gobbled up a superfluous amount of food before you begin to feel full, exceeding the body's needs and not leaving enough time for digestion or assimilation.

The Immune System – Our Line of Defence

Looking after our health successfully is a complex task. To help us, we're all equipped with a protector, the immune system, which is constantly battling against potential invaders, showing how incredibly important its role of defence is.

We will now go through the list of its troops and their roles. The first stronghold of the immune system is made up of the body's visible barriers. The skin, which resists the entry of micro-organisms, also secretes anti-microbial substances. Tears and mucus contain an enzyme that's capable of breaking down the cellular walls of bad bacteria. The saliva also contains antibacterial substances, and gastric acids provide a supplementary level of protection.

Certain bacteria, viruses and parasites succeed in getting beyond the first lines of the body's defence. Once they have entered the body, they face the internal immune system, which is able to identify and attack them. Viral and bacterial infections are the most common causes of illness. They will usually follow their course until the defence system puts up its guard by 'constructing' a specific immunity against each different type of virus and bacteria to destroy them, allow recovery and reduce the time of convalescence.

The immune system is, however, subject to some deficiencies: stress or neglecting your diet can soon destabilise it, leaving the path free to a series of extremely undesirable chain reactions that can cause illness.

Each illness wears out our immunity a little bit more, forcing changes in our metabolism, when genetic mutations and finally abnormal cellular growth can occur, which can sometimes be malignant and lead to cancer. The process is usually quite slow, taking many years and going through different pathological stages before becoming a diagnosed illness.

To maintain an efficient immune system is therefore a high priority in order to minimise the frequency and seriousness of illness.

Ageing – A Programmed Evolution

The ultimate and major common denominator among all human beings is the progressive deterioration of our vital functions. Fundamentally linked to our lifestyle, ageing has a dark side that slowly and inescapably imprints deterioration on various tissues until there ceases to be any cellular and respiratory activity at all.

This deterioration is felt bit by bit from the age of 35. From this time in our lives, our capacities tend to diminish – starting with our digestive and hormonal abilities – and they register more pronounced slowing on a seven-year cycle: 35, 42, 49, 56, 63, 70, 77. These stages require us to readjust our food to coincide with the decline in our capacities. To behave like a responsible adult, we must take this slowing down of our metabolism into account and act according to our age. The quality of how we age is dependent on accepting this maturity.

No single thing is responsible for ageing. Hormones certainly play a part as hormonal production slows, but the whole metabolism plays a part in ageing: our digestive abilities and the assimilation of food, diminishing cell regeneration and reduced capacity to slow down the natural oxidation process of our bodies. We are always the age of our organs, because genetics are a constant factor in the ageing process: for example, at the age of 66, even if we do well in a check-up, the vital organs – the liver, heart and stomach – are still all 66 years old. If we don't take this into consideration when making lifestyle decisions, then we increase our chances of premature ageing.

Nevertheless, ageing is due to a decrease in the quality of protein reproduction, and this accounts for a vast area of investigation that we're working on at the Academy of Biontology. While we look into it, we can be sure of one thing: the more we age, the more laborious it becomes for us to extract proteins from food that we must then break down to make our own proteins, containing our tissular and genetic identity. At the same time, the ageing body's capacity for absorption, like our ability to digest, both weaken. And this decline in protein renewal has repercussions on the quality of our bones. This is why osteoporosis threatens some of us as we get older.

Food, Our Source of Health

So, good engineering and a choke are enough to make the engine start – but you also need petrol, and not just any petrol. The body's petrol is food.

Through the centuries, Chinese medicine has

studied the workings of the human body and passed down an experimental knowledge and a precise analysis of the relation between food and health. Its conclusions are confirmed by modern scientific observations: a good working body relies on nutrition, which itself can be largely responsible for the ability to combat illness, ageing and, indirectly, life expectancy.

From the food we consume and the substances we produce, our bodies are constantly changing in structure, harnessing their own energy to carry out their functions and cause essential biochemical transformations: brain activity, the heartbeat, breathing, digestion, limb movement and the combination of 'functional' molecules, such as enzymes, hormones and neurotransmitters.

During digestion, the intestine will only keep whatever is useful to it. This conversion of food into nutrients means waste is rejected through the stools, while the nutrients head towards the cells. This is a journey that must constantly be prepared for, so that the nutrients don't end up going on a detour or the wrong way. This shows the pivotal role of digestion and the important role of the intestine.

So, what does the body really need? The three essential nutrients are proteins, lipids and carbohydrates. We have to assimilate these three nutrients in the right proportions in order to adequately feed our billions of cells, develop the reserves of what we consume for when our bodies find themselves in need, and release the necessary energy for metabolism. It's vital to understand that these basic elements of nutrition must be consumed every day, even if the body shows foresight by setting aside certain substances.

Proteins make up the cornerstone of the body; they see to the vast majority of cellular functions. About 15 per cent of what we consume should be proteins, and it's vitally important to respect this necessary ratio. It should be a balance of vegetable and animal proteins.

Lipids are fats that the body stores in reserves, and they represent around 30 per cent of our daily food intake. They make up a large part of the energetic realm of the body, allowing the transport of liposoluble vitamins A, D, E and K, and taking part in the development of many hormones.

For lipids, as for proteins, they should be vegetable-based and mainly unsaturated fats. However, animal-based fats are important in small doses, because they see to the maintenance of cells and the nervous system.

Good lipids – fatty unsaturated acids – can be

divided into sub-groups: omega 3, omega 6 and omega 9. The daily requirement for omega 6 is around 1.5g, and 0.5g for omega 3. At present, the recommended amount of omega 9 is unknown. Omega 3 is often removed from food today when it is processed – a regrettable move because omega 3 carries out the synthesis of certain hormones, namely the sexual and tissular ones. Sixty per cent of the brain is made up of fatty matter; isn't that a great reason to increase our intake of good lipids in food?

About 45 per cent of our intake should be devoted to carbohydrates – that's about 100 to 150g a day, regardless of body weight. Carbohydrates are the essential source of energy production, they help to maintain the structure of the conjunctiva (the transparent mucous membrane that covers the white of the eye), and the cells of the nervous system feed exclusively on them. Those carbohydrates with a slow absorption rate – called complex carbohydrates – are distributed to the cells in a prolonged and progressive way, sustaining the body's energy from one meal to another. They most notably have the advantage of being an excellent safeguard against hunger pangs.

Rapidly absorbed carbohydrates remain at the heart of a number of controversies. Some people avoid them at all costs because they make the glycemic load (the blood glucose levels) soar, yet there are some fast carbohydrates with a weak glycemic index that are the exception to the rule. Sugars and sweets are the subject of debate in our society among slimming aficionados; nevertheless, the glycemic index – which changed the way many think about nutrition – determines sugars and sweets as being of poor nutritional value.

As well as these nutrients, the body needs vitamins, trace elements and fibres. And let's not forget water, which is a priority, since it is our essential component, making up around 65 per cent of our weight. Our bodies obtain most of their 'new' water from the fluids that we drink and get about 20 per cent from food.

Vitamins are substances that are as varied as they are indispensable for multiple chemical reactions. Their attributes are identified under different letters of the alphabet and are divided into two groups: liposoluble (soluble in fats) vitamins A, D, E and K; and hydrosoluble (soluble in water) vitamins B and C. Exceeding the recommended amount of certain vitamins, such as A and E, can be dangerous. Also note that certain vitamins are only retained by the body if they are absorbed in the presence of another.

Another link in the food chain is trace elements

(minerals) which, even if they are consumed in small quantities, are indispensable to numerous metabolic, structural and functional tasks. Many are essential because the body cannot synthesise them, so we must therefore get them from food. They are unequally distributed among various types of food, in meat as well as vegetables. The daily requirements of minerals are so variable that they range from those stated in grams, such as sodium (Na), chlorine (Cl) and calcium (Ca), to those measured in microgrammes (a millionth of a gram), such as iodine (I), chromium (Cr) and selenium (Se).

Calcium and phosphorus (P) are used in the formation of bone and dental structure; sodium, chlorine, potassium (K), calcium, magnesium (Mg), sulphur (S) and phosphorous are involved in numerous processes, including the regulation of the acid base. Meanwhile, iron (Fe), important for haemoglobin, and iodine (I), important for the thyroid hormone, are involved in transporting oxygen and regulating energy. Other minerals help to revitalise enzymes that specifically work for the many metabolic and immune functions.

Alimentary fibres don't have a nutritional value to speak of and, moreover, are not digested. When they pass through the intestines, they help to maintain a good transit of food. Thanks to their powers of water absorption, alimentary fibres improve the volume of the bolus and the consistency of stools, stimulating the intestine's contractions and supporting the colon's bacterial activity. Another asset is that they demand slow chewing, which is a good 'cosmetic' reason to eat less, as the feeling of fullness can regulate the appetite before greed starts to override our physiological needs.

Proteins, lipids, carbohydrates, vitamins, trace elements, fibres: in order to consume the correct amount, it's worth familiarising yourself with these suppliers of health. We must help our bodies, as, if we don't, sooner or later they will rebel, notching up illness on their journeys and thus reducing our shelf lives. But don't get too scared: if, day by day, we consider our individual resources and respect the hazards of our age, we can get stronger and lead happier, longer, healthier lives.

CHAPTER TWO

YET EVERYONE'S DIFFERENT

We've just been looking at the similarities that make the human machine a 'manufactured model'. At the same time, however, there are many characteristics that make every one of these models individual. There isn't one unique model, but millions of different ones with obvious disparities.

Each to Their Profile

All you have to do is look at the physical aspect of each person to face the facts: our bodies present indisputable similarities but also obvious unique characteristics: one has brown hair, the other blonde; one measures 1.6m in height and the other is extremely tall. It's our hereditary background that determines these characteristics, by means of a distinctive and permanent sign: DNA, our genetic code.

The fact that our outward appearance differs from one individual to another has little impact on the activity and metabolism of our bodies. On the other hand, the variants brought about by the genetic code influence our functional capacities and create specific responsibilities for each of us for the duration of our lives.

Another thing that varies from one person to another is the quality of the 'terrain' (or acid-base equilibrium) and the body's main vital functions: resistance of the immune system and the ability to assimilate food, which is sometimes limited by intolerances of varying severity. One may find it harder than another to regulate its 'terrain', while one will be more gifted at producing free radicals (which are involved in the prevention of cell damage). Sensitivities and similarities combine, honing themselves as time goes by to form taste, adding a troublesome variant to the complexity of nutrition: the whims of cravings.

Finally, age and weight are additional factors that adjust our physical appearance and weigh down our physiological state in a complex way. Because of genetics and a range of functions, and because of overconsumption and, at times, age, different individuals will put on a bit or a lot of weight, while others put on only a little, or none at all.

Each to Their Genetic Code

Each human being is unique. We can resemble each other, but our genetic code differentiates us from all other living beings. The genetic code, DNA (deoxyribonucleic acid), contains the set of precious information that is necessary for our development. We find it in every single one of our cells, because, when they feed themselves while filling with proteins, they pass on this code to the entering protein, thanks to a natural process of breakdown and reconstitution. As a consequence, we possess unique digital codes, unique blood analyses, which integrate the major information of this code.

This genetic 'sticker' obviously has a large influence on our shape and our journey through life. It compulsorily determines a number of assets, handicaps, weaknesses and resistances which bind us together during our life. It can sometimes be disturbing to meet two people who have a similar composition, who eat in the same way, have the same job and live in the same area, but who have radically different profiles: one is thin, the other prone to chubbiness; one is a faithful devotee of sugar, without any glycemic responses, while the other suffers from stomach aches (evident from the light marks on their pale face). So the contradictions of the human body – and, indeed, the injustices linked to predetermined genetic inheritance – reveal themselves to us. It's up to us to adapt our lifestyle to suit our own personal inheritance.

Each to Their Terrain

Our 'terrain' is what's inside our bodies, and includes everything they're composed of. In short, it's our substance. We are expected to carry out four types of actions in this terrain, all indispensable to maintaining life within the body: acid reduction, alkaline oxidation, alkaline reduction and acid oxidation.

After swallowing food, the body must carry out two main operations: oxidisation and then reduction of this food. It's like burning a log. If you want to make the log hot, you have to add fire. As it burns and is consumed, it produces ash – that's what we mean by the reduction process. The same thing goes for our bodies: as we use the energy that we get from oxidised food, this food is reduced, leaving its 'ashes' as a residue.

However, the chemical reactions of oxidisation and reduction can only be carried out in an environment where bases (alkali) and acids are balanced. This is why our terrain must be an acid-reducer, acid-oxidant, alkaline-oxidant and alkaline-reducer. Depending on our genetic history and body type at birth, our ability to undertake these actions varies from one individual to another. So, for some, there will be less acid-reduction and more alkaline-oxidation. We're all predominantly one of the following: acid-reducing, acid-oxidising, alkaline-oxidising or alkaline-reducing – although we all possess a little of each of the other three. Each of us carries the substance that makes up every human in the world in our own personal way.

It's dangerous to change the nature of our terrain, as we risk it losing its ability to protect itself and expose itself to illness. And, if we change it too quickly for an environment that is too acid-oxidant – the cancer zone – illness becomes permanent.

The Four Territories

	ACID-OXIDISATION **Liver, gall bladder** Muscular problems Juvenile illnesses and viruses Fatty deposits	ALKALINE-OXIDISATION **Heart, small intestine** Circulation and inflammatory problems Surplus of free radicals
OXIDISATION		
REDUCTION	ACID-REDUCTION **Kidneys, bladder** Crystallisation, demineralisation Bone problems	ALKALINE-REDUCTION **Lymphatic circulation, lungs and large intestine** Oxygenation problems Fluid retention Territory of microbes, difficulties with blood circulation

Ph0   Acid   Ph7   Alkaline   Ph14

On the other hand, by staying within our terrain, and by carefully exercising the differences and properties they have inherited, our bodies can enjoy the use of their proper regenerative set-up. It's much better to adapt to our terrain, accommodate it and supply it with the appropriate nourishment. However, if the architecture and structure of the terrain are shaky, no matter what therapy we follow, there's nothing that can be done. The only way to rehabilitate our terrain is through preventative medicine.

How can we prepare our terrain? We have a base index at our disposal: the pH scale, which measures the degree of acidity or alkalinity of any substance. This index goes from 0 to 14: from 0 to 7 is declining acidity, 7 is neutral, and then from 7 to 14 alkalinity is on the increase.

The pH scale can be analysed by urine tests, and, faced with this information, we have another index, the PRAL (Potential Renal Acid Load). This is a scale that measures the acidifying power per 100g of food, and is scientifically determined by a blood analysis. (You can read more about PRAL in the ABC of Health, at the back of this book.)

Current indicative lists on the PRAL of food are available and allow us to eat more or less 'acid' as we please, according to our pH level, in order to re-establish the balance of our terrain's acid-base. For most of the time, however, we have to give priority to alkaline foods, for the very good reason that our bodies have a natural tendency to acidify as they function. They are constantly producing acidic waste. Moreover, 'modern' diets and their many excesses (such as drugs and additives) also make them more acidic.

Each to Their Tastes, Appetites and Ability to Assimilate

There's no accounting for taste. We know that our senses are changeable and we respond with a changing take on the outside world as we go through life. This gap between perception – as well as appreciation – and reality influences the affinities that we commonly call taste. Some of these affinities are opposed to others, and it's interesting to note that this finally confirms that, when it comes to our sense of taste or attractions, it's 'each to their own': some would sell their soul for sugar, others for salt, some for meat, or bread, cheese or pasta, etc. Again, it's each to their own. And also it's each to their own bad tastes and weaknesses – to the great detriment of our health, because sometimes we just eat too much harmful food.

Tastes develop as we age, because little by little our palate matures and our selection is widened by a constantly growing range of tempting popular dishes, which don't really help matters. The 'user-friendliness' gets into the mix, dressing up nutritious needs as pleasure, motivating a distinct tendency to make gourmet – rather than strictly healthy – dietary choices, or a mistaken feeling that we should be in professional or emotional agreement with others and therefore adopt other people's poor choices. Socially, or out of courtesy, we eat properly; out of friendship or complicity, we agree wholeheartedly with the excess dietary desires of our neighbours, friends or spouse until good sense re-establishes itself to make our tastes agree with our nutritional responsibilities.

Then there are particular dietary complaints when it comes to quantity – appetites according to our lifestyle, particular habits and specific stresses. The more the body is seeking something, the more it must consume, just as the hotter it is, the more thirsty it becomes – what could be more natural? Hereditary characteristics also create needs that are proportional to body type. We only have to look around us to see this in some people measuring 2m in height who are very broad shouldered, while others, measuring 1.6m, are very slim. Of course, the 'broad shouldered' might overdo it and fill up their plates more generously!

Levels of taste and of quantity vary for each person. But our tools of digestion can also vary in their efficiency. We could therefore have a good, or not-so-good, ability to assimilate food, or even a particular tolerance or intolerance when it comes to certain foods. Adjustments are necessary so that our motor's horsepower can reach its full potential. It's up to each of us to make sure that we overcome its laziness and slowness.

To Each Their Intolerances

Weaknesses, a poor ability to assimilate, a lazy intestine – our tools of digestion and immunity can be more or less sharp when it comes to their mission. But some food makes our bodies, or parts of our bodies, suffer, and we call this type of complaint (which is sparked off by food itself) a 'food allergy'. It's up to us to watch what we eat and cut out substances that cause intolerance – another task that shows the importance of eating correctly.

These days, there are numerous tests that can tell us why we've had a hostile reaction to food, which makes it easier to provide corrective treatments. These mainly consist of totally cutting out the trigger food, without causing an imbalance in our diet. For example, if a particular food represented an important supply of protein, then it must be replaced by something else that has the same protein supply. The main intolerances are down to lactose and gluten contained in certain cereals and in eggs.

In order to better understand the phenomenon of food intolerance, we must remember that each time we eat food for nutrition – whether that's vitamins, minerals, carbohydrates, proteins or fatty acids (various types of fat) – whatever we're eating will possess precise characteristics and will require specific enzymes to break it down. An apple, for example, has its own enzymes, as does milk. The body therefore has to produce its own digestive enzymes, and it needs an innumerable range of them. We are currently aware of more than 100,000 different enzymes that break down different types of food; there are certainly more but we just haven't identified them yet. These enzymes are produced every day by the pancreas.

The process happens like this: when we consume something – let's say milk – as soon as it's in the mouth it is immediately analysed by receptors which, thanks to the tastebuds, inform the brain, which immediately triggers the production of a specific enzyme that can digest lactose and all the other constituent parts of milk. Some enzymes might already have a problem with their design from birth, and the number of defective enzymes tends to increase as we get older, at a time when they are supposed to be adapting to a change in our diet from milk to solids. Some are developed to digest breast milk before the teeth develop, but as the teeth (usually the incisors) push through and the child is able to cut, grind down and assimilate more solid foods, a number of other enzymes develop. Sometimes, from this point, the enzymes that are supposed to digest lactose are not produced. Lactose can no longer be digested by some people who, in theory, no longer need it.

What enzymes are required so that the mouth can analyse in partnership with the brain? This is where chewing becomes important, as it is the only factor likely to prompt the correct enzyme according to the flavours present in the mouth. Suppose that the enzymes programmed to digest a particular substance aren't as vigorous or numerous as they should be: the substance is correctly digested the first time, but the second less so, and not at all the third time, resulting in a flood of enzymes. In this scenario, the body instigates a food allergy, meaning that the substance in question cannot be broken down. Despite all the chewing, the acidity in the stomach and the bacteria in the intestine, only partial digestion is possible. These remaining unassimilated bits of food feed the bacteria and do not contribute to intestinal balance. If they aren't contained or reduced by these bacteria, they will proliferate and ferment (rot), which could lead to complications such as gastric ulcers, gastritis or type 2 diabetes.

To find out whether you're intolerant to a particular food, you need to do a test on the substance in question. Substrates of this food are mixed with the blood and then a simple test is conducted to identify any intolerances to it. When there is a reaction, there are various stages or levels of intolerance. As well as fermentations, symptoms of intolerance can range from a simple blocked nose, to fatty deposits and even tissue damage. As soon as you cut the food from your diet, there will no longer be reactions or side-effects.

The less intolerances are treated, the more likely it is that there will be significant damage, such as Hopkins syndrome and other degenerative illnesses. Much also depends on the individual's genetics and general level of wellbeing. We must realise that a food allergy is for life, and that any specific enzymes that we're lacking from birth will only reduce as we age. Some enzymes are a lot more fragile – those that digest red meat, for example, weaken as we get older – therefore we should eat less red meat the older we become.

At Merano, we are extremely vigilant when it comes to intolerance problems that can quickly disrupt the workings of our bodies, and we often cite the example of athletes who regularly stay with us to enhance their training. One ignored a range of allergies for years. We detected an intolerance to wheat – specifically to gluten. He was eating pasta and was suffering from a chronic inflammation of the intestine which caused a very high fermentation of undigested food. To feed him, we made him special peptides and proteins that were free of everything he was sensitive to. In other words, we were looking after his intestine first and foremost. After our intervention and alteration to his diet, the athlete could train successfully and he even won his category in the Olympic Games. To reiterate, by paying more attention to his weak points, we were able to reconcile him with his life and with himself.

To Each Their Age

Life is a giant puzzle, based on the same model for everyone, but made up of billions of pieces that are designed to personalise everyone's characteristics and flaws. As we progress through time, our weaknesses are often heightened. Everything is a matter of age – it's fate, and each time we talk about body weight and health, we need to take age into consideration. The ability to effectively metabolise food significantly diminishes with age. Logically, as time goes by, we should eat less, because the needs of our bodies change and we lose the ability to absorb food. As we age, we must rely on our intelligence and act to cut out any food we don't really need to eat.

To Each Their Diagnosis

It would be easier to look after our bodies if we were all designed according to a standard model, but we're not. Scientific studies and the development of our expertise at the Academy of Biontology have supplied us with an enormous amount of information and data about the workings of the human body. When we look after our health and wellbeing, we must bear this knowledge in mind, but we should never lose sight of the fact that individuals have affinities and unique characteristics. By treating each person according to a general model, we simplify the diagnosis and move away from reality.

In order to understand the physiology of each person and supply them with the adequate and necessary guidelines for their health and to advise them on a diet suited to their individual needs, we must, of course, consider their body shape. This is often a reflection of the state of their metabolism, but also the operation of their vital systems. These depend on a number of different criteria. None ever works in exactly the same way as their neighbour. Culture and history also play a determining role on our diet and the workings of our stomachs.

CHAPTER THREE

SOCIAL AND CULTURAL INFLUENCES

New social and cultural practices impose a number of nonconformities on our diet. For the past 40 years, we have seen much progress in many domains and it's undeniable that we live for longer and in better health than our ancestors did. However, all of this progress has been accompanied by significant changes in our behaviour, habits and tastes.

Lifestyles in Transformation

Between 1960 and 2000, the global population doubled. We must therefore find solutions to feed all these new mouths in a nutritious and efficient way. Our ancestors only had natural resources from fishing, hunting and gathering at their disposal. They stocked up with local agricultural produce because foodstuffs were rarely transported far from the site of production. This had its disadvantages: such a bland diet did not provide a sufficient mix of nutrients and led to deficiencies that caused numerous degenerative diseases. In some mountainous regions, for example, where cabbage was widely and frequently consumed, populations often suffered from iodine deficiency, which could lead to goitre and other thyroid problems.

Today, science has advanced in giant leaps when it comes to modes of transport, conservation, hygiene and product selection. It has also allowed cultures to diversify and enrich our culinary heritage. All of these have helped to improve the quality of our food. We have gained in terms of freshness, safety and variety; safety standards and scientific controls can guarantee hygiene. In our Merano laboratory, we pay maximum attention to all processed food, both in terms of hygiene and of diet.

On the other hand, the vast range of what we're offered to eat nowadays can have a negative impact when flavoursome – but also more sugary, salty, fatty and commercial – dishes seduce us at the expense of our health. We're offered increasingly sophisticated combinations of food which can easily start us on a spiral of excess. Likewise, the quest for a pleasing physique, in keeping with the demands of fashion and society, further distorts our understanding of a healthy weight. This requirement to be thin, in total opposition to the over-enhancement and high consumption of today's food, can cause excesses across the board: deficiencies, obesity, intolerance and allergies.

The modern technology that's applied to the food trade has completely changed our traditional rules of life, shifted our rhythms, unsettled our diets and created stress. In industrialised countries such as ours, these new habits are often out of sync with our true needs. We can do anything, swallow anything whenever, wherever and however we want to, without giving a single thought to the rules of nutrition and hygiene. But the consequences are unfortunate and it's getting harder and harder to find a way back to optimal nutrition and wellbeing.

The Overturning of Our Ancestors' Rules

What happened? In days gone by, women played a decisive role in preparing meals and organising the house. There was a strict, orderly and punctual time for meals: breakfast, lunch and dinner. The existence of such regularity deserved credit. Eating habits were passed from generation to generation; we ate according to our means, with the rhythms of the seasons governed by periods of sobriety and of celebration.

Today, in a society where families often break up and change, meal rituals have diminished and been replaced by people eating on their own, dislocated from the cornerstones of quality, punctuality and mutual conviviality. Women do less cooking – they have less time and less inclination to do so – and, quite frankly, men are often reluctant or unable to take it on. The passing on of knowledge and skills is now much less common, the rituals have diminished and been replaced by others less concerned with nourishment and communal experience.

At lunch, a new way of eating has been established: eating while working, hurriedly or perched on the edge of a table. Our era is one where the fast-food restaurant reigns supreme. It's true that we don't have enough time, that modern life is revealing itself to be more and more frenetic. However, it would be beneficial, in many respects, to give back to ourselves the means of organising and making meals in a rational way, to reclaim these rituals and fight against certain new rules and harmful habits, such as sandwiches, pizzas, hamburgers and other similar foods – even if this only means slightly improving the quality of these foods.

Women who have problems with their figure, or anxiety issues, have a tendency to skip lunch or they will have a nutritionally unbalanced meal such as just fruit or salad with, at best, a yoghurt, which paves the way for deficiencies and cravings. The vast majority of people who live in towns and cities eat what they can find, or what is offered to them, quick and ready-made, at the local cafe or in the work canteen, without worrying too much about its quality. And, if we were to ask people who usually eat their meals away from home whether they'd prefer to actually eat at home, 90 per cent would respond with: 'No, we don't have the time and we prefer to eat with our colleagues, going to a restaurant and chatting with them.' Worse, we also often hear people say that they just grab a quick bite to eat while on the move.

Yet when we eat, it's important to think of what we're in the process of doing, to give ourselves enough time and not to rush, and to be sitting down. It's vital that we chew, that we soak food with our saliva and that we never swallow anything whole. If we don't take these precautions, the absorbed food will be badly assimilated and diverted from its intrinsic purpose: to feed the body. Without this essential job, food will become waste more easily and will join the fatty masses that sooner or later all add up on the scales with potential fatal consequences: an increase in weight, little by little, until the day that a simple kilo too many may cause serious or even life-threatening health problems.

The Over-industrialised Food Processing Industry

New industrial manufacturing processes have changed the nature of the traditional diet landscape, transforming basic food such as bread, pasta and rice, among others. The quality of bread and pasta has changed in just a few years; manufacturers include additives in order to reduce cooking time, and they have become less good for our health.

Let's take milk as another example. Its quality depends on the conditions in which the cow was raised, which have generally deteriorated worldwide. Furthermore, 20 or so years ago, we would consume it as a drink, a cheese or a yoghurt. But these days it has become king, contributing to the preparation of ready-made and easy-to-eat by-products: creams, ice creams, frozen yoghurts, chocolate bars and milky drinks which contain such a multitude of artificial ingredients that the end products are far removed from the wholesome original substance.

And we consume so much of it. All you have to do is cast an eye over the supermarket shelves, and you'll see that items containing milk occupy almost a third of the whole area. But what we're swallowing is not really milk: it's enriched milk, with more sugar and more this and more that, and it ends up being an eminently complex product that is very different from milk in its raw form.

Anyway, from now on we should question the role that milk plays in our diet. It's not easy to digest because it contains lactose, and, contrary to generally accepted ideas, it is not a significant source of easily absorbed calcium.

Another drawback of this age of overconsumption is that the food industry takes advantage of things such as food colourings, additives and flavour enhancers. We consume them together with sweetening agents which are sneaked into numerous industrially manufactured products. Everything is done to intensify productivity, break use-by date records and please the palate. And why not? The only problem is that our health takes a battering.

It's up to us as consumers to make good choices and go for natural food whose original quality is preserved, rather than food that's been modified.

Ready-made Food

A large number of restaurants now use pre-prepared food. Some chefs play with flavours to please our palates, so that a dish wins the approval of people who would rather appreciate a good taste over quality ingredients.

It's even worse in the world of fast food, where fat, sugar and salt are used liberally because they provide the 'scent' to dishes to make them more appealing. Tough luck for the body that is tempted. It's hardly surprising that there has been such an increase in obesity in developed countries where this kind of food is widely available.

Mass retailers offer pizzas, various dishes with a wide range of sauces and refined basic ingredients. Even some simple salads are gently and sophisticatedly supplemented with sugar and fat, in order to cheaply titillate the tastebuds. These dishes are consumed out of laziness: there's no need to prepare them. They can be eaten quickly (and badly) at the drop of a hat: in front of the television, standing up or on the telephone, without even bothering to sit at the dining table, and therefore interfering with the time that should be dedicated to meals.

Many people who work say that they don't have the time to cook, nor even to think about it. They buy things that are ready-made, or only need a few minutes to prepare; they eat the same dishes in the canteen at their place of employment. Not to mention those people who use the microwave to quickly reheat pre-prepared meals, or hastily make TV dinners that go against nutritional guidelines.

Fresh produce is a world away from these ready-made dishes. We should frequently opt for frozen food such as plain vegetables picked then packed without additives of any kind or fish which is frozen and packaged where it is caught. Such foods have a high nutritional value.

The Dangers of Snacking

The number of individual products in the food industry is overwhelming everyone and is leading to the destructive phenomenon of snacking. This is something that young people particularly succumb to, as they are more sensitive to taste than quality.

It's easy to prove this – just leave them to make their

own meals and you'll see a strong temptation to open the cupboard and reach out for chocolate bars, crisps, biscuits, snacks and other nightmare foodstuffs that can be quickly guzzled down. They can get into the habit of eating tempting snacks at whatever moment, filling up with various flavours, sugars and added fats – behaviour that does not engender a healthy diet. It's important to remember that the brain activates the appetite, as well as giving the signal of being full about 15 or 20 minutes after the start of the meal. So, when snacking increases the number of mealtimes we have, these signals are disturbed.

Thrift and Speculation, to the Detriment of Food

It's clear that production costs have changed the quality of food. A farmer who rears rabbits, chickens or cows in a non-intensive manner will feed them appropriately and will get a far superior quality of protein in the meat compared to if they were farmed intensively. At the supermarket, the difference between intensively farmed chickens and those traditionally reared is obvious: their price goes from cheap to three times as much for added value. This would suggest that we have to make a financial choice between eating healthily with good-quality food and sacrificing this to spend more on other things in our lives.

A Global Food Trade

Borders no longer exist. Societies are becoming more multiracial and multinational. A sign of this globalised time is that we can find everything everywhere: in every city we can buy specialities from Japan, from China, from India, from South Africa. Equally, the supermarkets in developed countries are full of international produce. This additional supply is pleasing, even if its diversity can interrupt the coherence of a consistent, homogenous diet.

Shortages and Excesses

All these factors contribute significantly to nutritional deficiencies and extremes. This dietary imbalance can lead to excess weight and declining health. To satisfy the body, we must give it a daily supply of a certain amount of proteins, carbohydrates, fats, vitamins, trace elements and water, with a good ratio of each of these elements (see the Nutritional Requirements section in the ABC of Health, at the back of this book).

Carbohydrates are the main enemy. Eaten in excess,

they risk not only enriching the fatty tissues, but also increasing the blood's glycemic index and affecting the body's metabolism.

Down With Sugars!

What are the effects of all these dietary changes? Excess weight, for sure, but also obesity, hypertension, cholesterolaemia, and sometimes sterility and impotence for some men. Young people, of course, have a resistance which can help to curb the bad effects of today's behavioural habits and regain their health. But, from the age of 35, it's a little more difficult, and by the age of 50 it's even harder.

Going back in time may appear to be unachievable. However, we shouldn't just think that there's nothing we can do. On the contrary, it's all about becoming aware of things in a new light, appreciating the stumbling blocks and proving that, with a bit of vigilance, knowing how to take control of yourself and feeding yourself a little or a lot depending on interdependent needs (such as your normal level of activity, job, family history) can be achievable and enjoyable. When your needs change, your habits – the good ones, that is – must follow!

CHAPTER FOUR

HUMANS AND WEIGHT

'Good' weight isn't about what most of us believe it to be, i.e. aesthetic criteria. In many cases, fluctuations in weight are down to health problems of varying degrees of seriousness. An unbalanced diet doesn't always mean a gain in weight – for many of us, it can cause an accumulation of fat; for a few others, it can manifest itself through other serious problems. These problems are often apparent physiologically, such as in the deposit of crystals that permeate tissues and joints. In a case such as this, there isn't an obvious gain in weight, but there are consequences that can be dangerous for our health.

At the start of our lives, we don't seem to differ much from each other; however, we are all born with predispositions that could weigh heavily on the scales for the whole of our lives. Individuals are determined by their genetic code. This inheritance, which goes back seven generations, predetermines conditions such as portliness, which can in turn lead to other problems. So certain people are thin and stay that way, while others are genetically disposed to being fatter.

What do we mean by the expression 'to put on weight'? When and how do we influence what the needle on the scales points to, when it should ideally remain at around the same point from a particular age?

Body Weight

Our body weight is comprised of a number of distinct substances: the weight of the fluids which make up our bodies (around 16–18 litres) and the weight of our organs, which will remain at around the same weight when we're adults, no matter who we are. This is not the case for bone density, muscular mass or fat density, which vary according to the individual.

Genetic factors influence the unique composition of the body, and how balanced each person is in terms of their bone, muscular and fatty masses. We can, for example, be tall and slender and have more weight in fat, or be short and stocky and have a larger muscle or bone density. This is because there can be thin and thick skeletons, which vary in weight. And, when it comes to problems regarding the skeleton, unsurprisingly we can't do much about it except to check the level of harmony between these three major components of our bodies.

So, when we think about gaining or losing weight, it's very important to keep the body's composition in mind: fat, muscle and bone.

Deadly Adipocytes

If the weights of different body masses make up the individual structure of a person's body, then their ultimate weight is usually determined by the body's fat mass. Adipocytes, also known as lipocytes or fat cells, are the cells which inflate as they absorb and store fats. From birth, we possess a given number of fat cells – this varies from one individual to another depending on their genetics. They are mainly situated behind the superficial layer of the supporting tissue, the epidermis. Depending on the person, there can be 30–60 billion.

During growth, these fat cells multiply and reach 300 billion for some people. Their number settles definitively from the onset of puberty, determining the density of fatty tissue in the body for the rest of our lives. Between childhood and adolescence, if we have botched up our 'dietary homework', we will find ourselves overweight from the moment of puberty, when the definitive number of adipocytes stabilises. What's more, these adipocytes will never disappear. The number of them will always remain the same, but, if we lose weight, they will become smaller, reducing their volume.

Each adipocyte can accommodate more than 29 times its volume of fat. This knowledge alone can have a detrimental effect on our bodies – it can sometimes lead to parents handing down a string of physical troubles and bodily dysfunctions to their children. Add to this the dangerous and powerful growth in childhood obesity, which has serious repercussions for the whole of adult life, and you'll understand why it's important to understand more about the constitution of the human body.

Why Losing Weight is Irrational

Why do we want to lose weight? That's the one question that people obsessed with weight loss never seem to ask themselves. An unhealthy supply of food can sometimes lead to fatty tissue tripling, quadrupling, or increasing even more. Fine, say the obsessives, we'll deprive ourselves of it, we'll cut down our food intake. However, they are wrong, and they seem to be unaware that, in addition to the amount of food we eat, its quality, effective assimilation, good digestion, proper breakdown and correct elimination as waste must all be taken into account.

By throwing ourselves into the spiral of slimming diets, which are usually unbalanced and nutritionally meagre, we deprive our bodies of vital elements. The result can also be disappointing – we often notice an increase in weight by dint of recurring diets.

Let's take the protein-rich diet. It results in a rapid weight loss, but the fatty mass – which is the most difficult to get rid of – only decreases a little (at best, 30g to 40g a day). On the other hand, this diet wears down the bone mass and muscular mass because, to take back what it's owed, the body starts to eat the proteins in its own muscular structure and the minerals in its bone structure. The result is that, without realising, followers of this diet lose less fatty mass and more muscle and bone density, which is likely to lead to serious problems such as osteoporosis.

Good and Bad Fats

Excess fats have different causes, different effects and different locations, and diet isn't always solely to blame. But everyone has a certain sensitivity to one manifestation or another of adiposity, and we are all likely to face an issue with our weight at some time. Excess fats are undesirable because their effect on our physical appearance doesn't tally with current ideas of what is attractive. It would be wiser, however, to look at the damaging effects that these fats have on our health rather than just concentrating on what we see in the mirror. Looking after your weight throughout your life is first of all about eliminating the bad side-effects of fat, without thinking about the difference it makes to our appearance. To achieve this, we must firstly identify the origins of weight gain and understand the location of fats that have already formed. We must then consider good and bad fats.

It is possible to identify four different sorts of fats: fats of a glycemic origin, fats due to overeating, stress-related fats and fats due to hormones. The first two are the worst for our health. We must also look at fats that emerge as we get older.

Glycemic Fats

These are mainly due to an overconsumption of carbohydrates, notably fast carbohydrates (refined sugar and white flour). What happens when we eat too many fast sugars? The body triggers off a supply of insulin via the pancreas in order to transform the carbohydrates into fat. But, when there is too much, the insulin remains in the fat cells. During this time, the brain finds itself lacking carbohydrates – hypoglycaemic – and asks for more when it has actually already had too much.

Worse, this second dose of carbohydrates causes a new insulin reaction and another accumulation of fat. This then deposits itself on the periphery and the inside of the body, which will eventually cause the appearance of a large amount of fat around the tummy and – more dangerously – around the organs and major blood vessels, which can signal major health risks.

To turn things around, we need to be patient in order to radically modify the terrain and reset our biological clocks. This takes around nine months, the duration of a pregnancy. We'll see in the following chapter how to regulate the desire for sugar and bring the glycemic index under control.

Fats Due to Overeating

Fats due to overeating derive from ingesting too much food – and in particular too much of the wrong sort of food. The surplus of food leads to the production of these kinds of overeating fats. This type of fat can also be identified in the other three fat categories. They are linked to an erratic diet – eating too much of everything. Over-calorific food that is too fatty, too sugary and too salty; eating frequently, abundantly and unsystematically; genetic predispositions; and a lack of physical activity are all behind accumulating fats by eating too much.

The effects of this excess load are clear to see. Too many kilos of fat in the body have grave effects on the health: cardiovascular disease; gastro-hepatic, kidney, vein, bone, breathing and joint problems; and a reduced life expectancy. Not to mention psychological issues of low self-esteem from the impact of social attitudes about heavy people.

An established excess weight can lead to obesity, with levels going from light to extremely severe. However, true obesity is not detected by an excess of weight, but of fat. This curse, which tends to develop in Western countries, affects both sexes and all generations, and increasingly children, teenagers and the elderly.

When we know that each day we can only lose around 30g to 50g of pure fat at most, and if, for an average of 40g, we're only losing 14.6kg of pure fat a year, you can only imagine the goodwill, patience and medical support that losing this weight will require.

Fats Due to Stress

Stress, the 'scourge of the century', is a devious phenomenon, and its consequences are often reflected in our appearance.

The seriously 'stressed' have significant needs for corticoids and adrenalin, usually regulated by the suprarenals, two small glands that can be found above the kidneys. These work with two other hormones, insulin – secreted by the pancreas, and whose impact we have already seen – and hormones produced by the thyroid, which can speed up a heart attack.

The more stressed we are, the more we seek these suprarenals, and when they work the thyroid does as little as possible. When the thyroid is in hypofunction, our metabolism slows down. This means it consumes less and creates superficial abdominal fats below the navel, which, although they are far less dangerous than those due to too many carbohydrates, are just as unsightly. So we can suffer either hypo- or hyperthyroidism. The first has a tendency to make you fat, the second to make you thin.

There are several antidotes to stress. Physical activity is recommended, but we must nevertheless be aware that too much exercise can also lead to stress. Meditation is a fantastic option. We can also overcome disturbance linked to stress by taking the proper time out during meals. Often people who are stressed will eat quickly, not taking much notice of what they are swallowing, and not chewing properly. Wolfing things down means the receptors in the brain remain impassive and don't register that we are eating. So, instead of one portion, we might have two, even three. We swallow more than we need, and we're very likely to digest these large quantities badly and to stockpile the surplus.

To get rid of these excesses we must take the time to chew; the brain can therefore see when it has had its correct ration of carbohydrate and nutrients, and tell us we are full.

Fats Due to Hormones

Hormonal fluctuations, which have a large influence on the metabolism, can also have an effect on the weight of fats. Hormones secreted by the thyroid are particularly involved here, capable of either accelerating or slowing down the activity of the heartbeat, the bloodflow and the energy produced by the human body, which has to remain at 37∞C. Evidently, when these functions slow down, we burn less. Getting rid of the surplus, the leftover bits of food, becomes an impossible mission for the body and, fatally, we stockpile more and more fats, particularly around the hips, thighs and bottom.

Thyroid problems can be down to genetics, causing small problems which get worse as we grow older. Illness would imply that the body needs therapy, but, before talking about illness, we need to examine the main signs of the problem – a blood test will help to evaluate the condition and its context, and treat symptoms with full knowledge of the cause.

There is another link between weight and hormones: taking the contraceptive pill, which, when it's poorly prescribed or at the wrong dosage, can lead to an imbalance of progesterone and oestrogen, leading to significant adiposities.

The location of fats

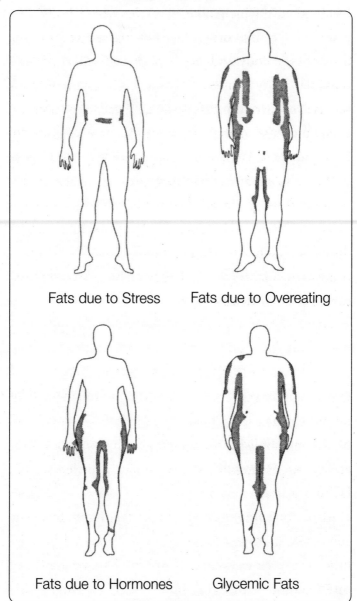

Fats due to Stress

Fats due to Overeating

Fats due to Hormones

Glycemic Fats

If excess weight is accompanied by an increase in non-localised fats which take over the whole body, fats from a glycemic origin deposit themselves on the inside of the body and its periphery, in both curvy and muscular body shapes. Fats due to stress mainly fix themselves around the stomach and the bottom, sometimes also higher up the body, on the stomach, bust and arms. Depending on their origin, all of these visible and unattractive fats present health risks, ranging from a simple excess weight to a slowing down of the vital functions, and include severe diseases such as hypercholesterolemia, hyper-triglyceridemia, type 2 diabetes, hypertension and cardiovascular disease.

Fats Due to Ageing

Our weight changes with age, and it is even dependent on our age as ageing involves a general slowing down of the metabolism, which progressively reduces our ability to assimilate and eliminate nutrients, and favours water retention.

Also, don't forget our biological patterns: from the age of 35, a change in weight is accentuated little by little, every seven years. So putting on weight will often come hand in hand with ageing. This indisputable factor must be considered when we try to understand weight.

As we get older, we need to progressively cut down our daily food intake and follow recommended advice such as eating balanced and regular meals made of good-quality food, chewing for long enough and dedicating sufficient time to enjoy meals.

Of equal importance are the significant changes in the body's make-up between the ages of 20 and 70. We observe a natural reduction in muscular mass or a fall in bone density that accompanies a progressive growth in fatty mass. This can explain the problem of osteoporosis, which is linked with ageing.

Loss of Weight – Loss of Fats

For many reasons that we have been investigating, fatty mass is something that's on an upward trend. Firstly, we blame food, quite rightly, because for the most part it's responsible for weight gain. We could get thinner by cutting our food supply, or by rebalancing it, but the body doesn't like eliminating surplus fat and so will only do it sparingly and slowly. Adipocytes, in effect, will reduce in volume but much more slowly than the rate at which they are gained. They can fill again, and all the more so because their ability to extend is buoyed by a supply of lipids, or more carbohydrates or alcohol, which are then transformed into lipids. Somewhat reassuringly, it is impossible to gain 1kg of fat in a day.

Sometimes we can put on weight through an increase in muscular mass – this is proven by very sporty people. But when it's a question of what to lose, it's exclusively and invariably about losing fats, without wearing down the muscular or the bone mass. At Merano, we insist that, when you want to lose weight, it's the *fats* you need to lose. When people say to me, 'I've lost weight', I always respond by asking, 'What kind of weight are you talking about?' Lots of people trying to get thinner have only one obsession when they get on the scales: the fateful needle that shows the number of kilos, without caring much about what it is they have really lost. That's a shame for their health.

And if these people know how to start a diet, then they must also know how to change at least one of their dietary habits responsible for any weight gain once the diet is over. If not, they're heading towards a life that's full of frustration and yo-yo dieting.

When we understand that weight gain is usually down to a diet with too much fat, sugar and salt, that's over-abundant or has an imbalance of proteins, lipids and carbohydrates, and is often poorly distributed throughout the day, there is a choice to make between definitive weight loss or following bad habits. Too many diets, particularly if they've been followed for a long time or repetitively (such as those that favour proteins), cause regrettable deficiencies that can greatly harm the muscular mass and bone density, which will each deteriorate a lot more readily than fats.

If a person's eating pattern involves going without for a period of time, and then adopting another almost identical diet, this is inadequate. With this kind of attitude, there can only be losers: the more you lose, the more you put back on, and it becomes more and more difficult to lose the weight again. Then there are the associated health problems.

Instead of wanting to lose weight at all costs, it's much better to modify our diet, to try new rules and different behaviour, while always respecting our individual characteristics, and to take another look at these routines on each life cycle.

This is the only significant and basic advice that we need in order to be in harmony with our bodies. Of course, the results may be slower, but they will guarantee good health. In all cases, we should change our method of nutrition according to our genetics, our age and our professional and private life.

The Ideal Weight?

In order to size up our bodies and determine how much excess weight they have, there is one main approximate benchmark, the BMI, or Body Mass Index, a simple calculation between our height and our weight. All we have to do is divide our weight (in kilos) by our height (in metres) squared. The result is a value which can serve as a main reference for us when considering lifestyle changes that will lead to weight loss. If the number is between 19 and 23 for a woman, and between 20 and 25 for a man, then the weight is acceptable, and considered normal. For all those with a BMI over 25, we start talking about being overweight, and then, from 30 onwards, obesity.

This index does not take the bones or the muscles into account. To get additional information on any potential imbalance between the muscular, bone and fatty mass, which could lead to trouble with proper functioning of the body, we also need to know the percentage of fat. This is calculated by a procedure called a bioelectrical impedance analysis that we carry out for all of our patients, or by an impedancemetry balance. An impedancemetry balance is a method used to estimate body composition. It measures the impedance, or resistance, to an electrical signal as it travels through water in the body muscle and fat. The resistance is used to calculate the body fat.

By combining the results of the BMI and the percentage of fatty mass, we can work out and obtain a good reading of how the three masses are distributed.

Fatty mass makes up around 25 per cent of the total weight of a medium-sized young woman, and around 15 per cent of the total weight of a medium-sized young man. But a good state of health isn't automatically reserved for those who are thin rather than those who are larger. Being underweight logically involves a poor and harmful diet, with various deficiencies and various effects depending on the individual: hormonal problems, poor resistance, weak bones and wasting muscles.

The right weight does exist, but only if we understand how to lead a healthy life, without abuse, stress, unhealthy food or overeating. Equally, a healthy lifestyle should include taking a decent amount of exercise. Once these conditions have been achieved, the right weight will then follow, according to the body type. Above all, it's about health and vitality.

We should stop deceiving ourselves – the ideal weight as promoted in many parts of the media does not exist, or not as we imagine, at least. There is no stereotypical weight, only an individual one that is harmonious when it's accompanied by the right factors, including an adequate, unregimented, unrestrictive diet. To keep our bodies in continuous good shape, avoid illness and extend our life expectancy, we should not focus on the weight of our dreams as an objective, but a weight that's right for our health and our character.

It's obvious that, to look after our weight, the balance of food consumed – adjusted according to our age and the state of our bodies – is an indisputable factor. Not to forget chronobiology, which contra-indicates snacking. As we have seen, snacking triggers digestion and makes the whole process much more laboured, changes the pH of our urine and increases acidity, which in turn contributes to acidosis and water retention, which is a source of weight gain.

Weights and Measures

We say down with these ridiculous standards according to which a person measuring a certain amount must apparently weigh a certain amount! BMI is only a marker which shows that a person of 1.68m should weigh 58kg. It would be fanciful to only consider this point of view without looking at the personal factors which make up each individual.

Let's take a specific example. A sporty person measuring 1.8m in height can easily weigh 90kg, without being fat; this is nothing surprising, it's only the muscular mass, and it isn't damaging at all if this is a bit high. Muscles are heavier than fats which, at an identical weight, will be more voluminous and damaging to health. On the other hand, being less active yet of the same height and weight will make a person too heavy. For them, the right weight is around 75–76kg.

Other examples speak for themselves. Look at this case: a 48-year-old woman who measures 1.72m in height and weighs 74.4kg. Standards indicate that she should weigh around 62kg, made up of 51.2kg of lean body mass, of which 36kg should be muscular mass. Then we need to add 15 per cent of fatty mass. So her correct weight should be in the region of 64kg. To reach this reasonable weight, she must lose 6kg of fatty mass.

By looking at her diet, if we notice that she is eating too many carbohydrates, we would ask her to cut them down. And if, at the age of 48, her metabolism works with 1,800 calories a day (we give the amount of calories to give an idea of the quantity and not the nutritional value), then we can justifiably recommend her to be careful, because in three years' time her metabolism will only need 1,400 calories. If she doesn't follow these recommendations, she could reach 78kg, or even 80kg by the time she's 54. Another factor should also be pointed out: as she approaches the menopause (which occurs at an average age of 51), she faces a large risk of losing her muscular mass, in favour of fatty mass. The ideal for her shape and her health should be to bring her weight of 74.4kg down to 64 or 65kg over a period of nine months.

Another example: a man measuring 1.68m in height weighs 90kg. Before diagnosing anything, it is crucial to look at his excess weight. Are the amounts of fat due to carbohydrates, hormones, stress or a predisposition to portliness? Is his diet a bit too rich? When we have evaluated all of this, we must then show him a new way to eat, and this has to last for at least seven years. Weight is not the only indicator; his body composition is just as important.

Another case: a man of 65, 1.68m in height and weighing 65.7kg. This isn't too bad on first sight – his weight appears to be good. But after diagnosis we see that his weight is composed of 20kg of fatty mass – which is 30 per cent of his entire tissue, when the ideal is 15 per cent (20–22 per cent maximum). It's possible that his excess weight is harming his bones and could lead to osteoporosis, which is common after a certain age. Even though he weighs a reasonable amount, this man must also look again at his diet and do physical exercise.

So the perception of weight is not just a story of scales, it's all about harmony between the major components of the body, in relation to our genetic heritage, our age, our diet and our health.

CHAPTER FIVE

THE RISKS OF AN UNSUITABLE DIET

So many illnesses could be avoided if we just knew how to feed ourselves properly. A good diet isn't the only reliable route to take but, in any case, it's something that we can control and correct for the better on a daily basis. By understanding the close links that exist between an unbalanced diet and common illnesses, we can effectively prevent some of the harm they do, rather than trying to heal them all.

An Unhealthy Spiral

We have to face the fact: people who eat badly are inflicting all sorts of damage and excesses on their bodies, which can put its proper functioning in peril.

When we treat a machine badly, our behaviour upsets its mechanisms, making them jam and clog up. By rendering their functionalities unsuitable and superficial, we expose our bodies to a range of dysfunctions that are likely to end up as diseases.

Of course, we can't blame everything on the food we eat, but, quite frankly, our good health largely depends on it. The quantitative and qualitative aspects of diet must also be taken into account. For example, we state that an increase in daily food rations can cause a rise in obesity. Dr Graham Colditz of the Harvard School of Public Health estimated that, if obese adults in America slimmed down to their correct weight, it would prevent 96 per cent of diabetes, 74 per cent of hypertension cases, 72 per cent of coronary diseases, 32 per cent of tumours of the colon and 23 per cent of tumours in the breast. These figures speak for themselves and must draw people's attention to the importance of adequate nutrition.

Wouldn't it be better to think twice before we indulge in too much or too unhealthy food if it means we could live a longer, calmer, healthier and more balanced life? It's undeniable that modern consumers are presented with unhealthy products and that some of their ingredients, particularly chemical agents in the form of preservatives, colourings, emulsifying agents and flavour enhancers, end up in the human body, with harmful effects, on both excess weight and general health.

As with every sophisticated machine, the performance and activities of our bodies demand our efforts to supply them with enough fuel. Sometimes it turns out that, far from listening to the brain, the body will override logic and lead itself towards undesirable disorders. Just as we know how to make a machine work, we have identified the origin of most episodes of physical illnesses that are often only observed when they no longer fall under our control.

We will now focus on the lack or surplus of food which threatens our health so often: for example, too many or too few carbohydrates; too much food irritating the intestinal flora, not enough to enrich it; or a diet that is too acidic or lacking antioxidants.

Too Many Carbohydrates

They may flatter the palate, but we must pay attention to the amount of carbohydrates that we consume. We should opt for slow- rather than fast-releasing carbohydrates, taking into account the notion of the glycemic index of food.

THE GLYCEMIC INDEX (GI)

The glycemic index lets us classify food according to its sugar content. This measurement is very useful in preventing weight gain, obesity and diabetes, because it specifies the ability of food, after absorption, to increase the level of sugar in our blood, on a scale of 0 to 100. A low GI is less than 50, a medium one between 50 and 70, and a high GI is more than 70. By eating more food with a low GI, our feeling of fullness comes more quickly and is more stable.

Once carbohydrates have been eaten, they raise the level of sugar in the blood. This brings about a rise in insulin, a buffering hormone. As we have seen, the higher the glycemic load in food, the more the body produces insulin and creates a desire for sugar, which makes the body dependent on it. We can get rid of this harmful discharge of insulin by cutting out the food with a high GI, which is responsible for our putting on weight, especially around the tummy.

Fats resulting from carbohydrates invite themselves into the fatty tissue. But this isn't the worst thing – they also find their way into the brain fats and, by oxidising them, can eventually cause brain fatigue and memory loss. According to some studies, fats from carbohydrates may even be precursors to Alzheimer's disease.

They also infiltrate the blood vessels and vital organs such as the heart, increasing the risk of cardiovascular attacks and type 2 diabetes, which has a dietary origin (as opposed to type 1 diabetes, which is hereditary). By disturbing the flow of insulin, we are flirting with the very real danger of becoming a diabetic.

Foods with a High GI

STARCH/CEREALS
White rice
Risotto
Potatoes
Chips
Crisps
Lasagne
Ravioli
Gnocchi

BREAD
White bread (all kinds!)
Sandwich loaves
Baguettes and rolls
Crackers

Breadsticks
Croissants
Brioche
Sticky buns
Pain au chocolat

BREAKFAST CEREALS
Refined cereals
Wholegrain cereals
Cereal bars

BISCUITS (all, from white or wholegrain flour)

PIZZA

FRESH AND DRIED FRUIT
Grapes (fresh or dried)
Melon
Fig (fresh or dried)
Dates
Prunes
Bananas (mature ones)
Mustard
Fruit syrup (in a can)
ALL FRUIT JUICE (even 100 per cent fruit varieties)

JAM AND MARMALADE (made from white sugar)
Sugar – white, cane, brown

Honey (only in small quantities)

Syrup of corn, wheat and glucose

Maltose (found in beer)

Glucose

Molasses

Too Few Carbohydrates

Cutting out carbohydrates altogether from our diet is not a good idea, because it causes gluconeogenesis: forced to satisfy its need for glucose, the body sets its own mechanisms to work by transforming lipids and proteins into consumable energy. If this becomes regular, the process will lead to a series of negative consequences: a reduction in the lean body mass, which means extra work for the kidneys, and the build-up of deposits which may be eliminated via the urine, but, in the process, raise the level of acid in the blood and cause dehydration and demineralisation.

Foods with a low GI

STARCH/CEREALS

Long-grain, brown and basmati rice (preferably cooked in a rice cooker)

100 per cent wheat or wholegrain pasta

(always cooked al dente in a small amount of water for 10 minutes)

Pasta from kamut, spelt wheat, wholegrain buckwheat (cooked al dente for 8 minutes)

Soya pasta

Cooked grains of spelt wheat, barley, quinoa, kamut, oats, millet, wholegrain bulgur wheat

BREAKFAST CEREALS

Muesli without sugar

Porridge

FRESH AND DRIED FRUIT

Apples (fresh or dried, without added sugar)

Pears

Plums (fresh or dried)

Oranges/mandarins

Apricots

Kiwi fruit

Strawberries and all fruits of the forest

Grapefruit

Cherries

Papaya

Jam and marmalade without white sugar (sweetened with fructose)

Avocado

Mango

ALL VEGETABLES (RAW OR COOKED)

ALL PULSES: haricot beans, lentils, peas, broad beans, soya beans

SEEDS: sunflower, flax, sesame, pumpkin

NUTS: hazelnuts, almonds, pine nuts

NATURAL YOGHURT, without added sugar

DARK CHOCOLATE (70 per cent cocoa)

AGAVE JUICE OR FRUCTOSE

It's worth noting that the GI of some vegetables, including carrots and beetroot, increases depending on whether they're cooked (+) or raw (–).

Too Much Aggressive Food for the Intestinal Flora

Feeding our bodies on a daily basis is a must. Most chemical digestion occurs in the small intestine, so it must be carefully looked after in order to maintain its vitality and its protective flora. The intestinal flora are inhabited by helpful living bacteria that operate on good terms with the intestine. This develops a sort of active barrier which drives back all the food that's still being broken down, and all harmful substances that arise from its decomposition.

Around 500 species of bacteria permanently protect the intestine, mainly in the large intestine, the final digestive meeting place. After they have chosen their permanent home, we must domesticate these residents in our bodies and secure their necessary space. Their overpopulation, as with their under-population, goes against the good health and condition of the digestive system.

A series of scientific studies serves to demonstrate that these bacteria have an extremely important role, guaranteeing the protective balance of the intestinal microflora. Their presence in processed foods is beneficial. Unfortunately, a certain amount of undesirable and incompetent guests, whose use has become quite excessive and unjustified over the past few years, reduce and could even wipe out the work of these hard-working resident bacteria in the intestine. These include antibiotics, sulphamides, corticoids, laxatives and sometimes the contraceptive pill. Food colourings, preservative agents and pesticides also risk influencing this balance over the short or long term, in a process we call dysbiosis. Some heavy metals, such as lead or mercury, are also very dangerous to intestinal bacteria. Parasitic flora also generate dysbiosis.

Psychological traumas and stress are also decisively associated with dysbiosis, but, again, it is food itself that plays the most important role when it comes to the breakdown of food and the maintenance of flora. Some food elements, such as flour and refined sugar, can destroy it, while others can be a great help, such as fibre in vegetables. As for gluten, this sticky protein is another troublemaker, and dysbiosis reinforces its damaging side.

So, why should we safeguard the internal ecology of the intestinal system? Because it's the headquarters of the immune system's sphere of activity, with its developed lymphatic network. To put it bluntly, the more the flora is affected, the higher the intestine's defensive powers, and we should take into account that its vital role is to keep the body in the best health.

Scientific research is constantly progressing and developing: the significance of the acid-base balance of tissues, and the dangerousness and virulence of free radicals in the body are just two recent discoveries. This knowledge should influence our behaviour and adaptation of nutritional strategies which – it's important to remember – help to regenerate the cells, the organs and the immune system.

A Lack of Antioxidants

Free radicals are molecules whose activity is an obvious cause of internal and external ageing. We're becoming more and more aware of their damaging effects and, luckily, of the various ways in which they can be a nuisance and how to combat this. Free radicals attack the DNA of cells they encounter, causing an ionic imbalance, their decline and then death through oxidative stress. But what are 'free' radicals?

The body is guarded by an arsenal of antioxidants that are ready to neutralise and even prevent the formation of free radicals. This arsenal forms after an episode of unusually strong oxidation, which can be due to diseases or foreign bodies that are difficult to reduce and eliminate. Without sufficient – or with weakened – antioxidants, the body cannot defend itself against the battalion of free radicals. This battalion gets bigger and bigger because of external attacks that increase its production: sunburn and exposure to UV rays, smoking, alcohol, stress, various pollutions. The molecules lose an electron and become disabled. They then steal their missing electrodes from neighbouring molecules, unbalancing them in turn, and so on. This continuous chain can only be stopped by an antioxidant.

All the body's cells are affected by oxidative stress, with the brain and immune system cells particularly sensitive. And, when these lipids are attacked by free radicals, we're faced with a specific oxidative process which leaves a residue of rancid fat molecules. This residue starts to then damage the cellular membranes, progressively shrinking the cellular structures until they are exhausted. It's all the more unfortunate because fat drawn from food contains important liposoluble vitamins and essential fatty acids that the blood transports around the body in specific vehicles, called lipoproteins. In their original state, these are pretty inoffensive, but they can become very dangerous to the arterial walls when they are altered. Some lipoproteins with a low density – LDLs – transport cholesterol, so it's important to keep a watchful eye on them.

Too Much Acidity in Food

The acid-base relation is a fragile balance between alkalinity and acidity in tissues which must constantly be maintained. We should never underestimate its influence on the risk of serious metabolism problems.

Investigative methods and leading biotechnology give us access to a precise analysis of acidity or alkalinity in bodily fluids. The means of measuring is through the pH scale, going from 0 (total acidity) to 14 (total basic/alkalinity). Observing the breakdown of food during its combustion reveals the presence of enzymes that can adapt the digestive level of the ingested food, making it more alkaline, or more acidic, in order to optimise its assimilation. They can even evaluate the amount of waste products – alkaline or acidic – during this assimilation. It goes without saying that we should distinguish between acidic and alkaline food in order to maintain a correct pH level. Also, we shouldn't eat food that requires an acid medium (such as starchy food or carbohydrates) with food requiring a more alkaline medium (such as proteins) at the same time.

Tissues have an unfortunate tendency to increase in acidity, becoming very sensitive to chronic acidosis at the same time. This acidosis activates the ageing process, making the area fertile for the proliferation of germs of all kinds – bacteria, viruses and fungi. It also encourages the development of many diseases, from kidney and bladder problems to rheumatism, diabetes, hyperthyroidism and even cancer. Faced with this string of threats, even if food isn't the exclusive cause of acidity in the body, its contribution is such that we really should cut down the amount of acidic food we consume.

Furthermore, we must pay attention to an often hostile protein: animal protein, from red meat in particular. As soon as it's eaten, it produces uric acid – a real nuisance, containing substances that are extremely difficult to break down. To get rid of it, the blood cunningly deposits it in some tissues in the form of minuscule, but damaging, needles – monosodium urate crystals (MSUs). These help to initiate the acidification process, where we must be wary of the development of chronic acidosis. The more purines food contains, the more uric acid it creates, until it saturates the blood. When its presence in the bloodstream exceeds 70mg per litre, the situation becomes worrying as hyperuricaemia could occur.

Some tissues are fooled more easily than others into being impregnated by uric acid: cartilage, tendons and ligaments (which have fewer blood vessels), or those in colder parts of the body, such as the ears. An MSU deposit causes deterioration and precedes osteo-articular illnesses such as rheumatism, rheumatoid arthritis, osteoarthritis and tendonitis, or problems such as gout, sciatica, neuritis and the formation of kidney stones, gallstones and hepatic stones. When the MSU crystals deposit themselves in the central and most important joints, as in the tissues of organs including the kidneys, we have to worry about cases of chronic gout. It goes without saying that it would be wise to watch out for the precursory symptoms: chronic tiredness, feelings of nervousness, muscular pains, constipation, digestive problems, weak nails with the appearance of white marks, a coated tongue, acidic sweating with itchy eyes and mouth, chronic urinary and vaginal inflammations, acidic gastritis and colitis, with a bloated stomach or stomach cramps.

Acidosis is largely linked to demineralisation, because, as the blood becomes more acidic, the body uses its own means of protection to 'buffer' itself from the harmful effects of acidic blood. The body gets minerals – phosphates, calcium, magnesium, whatever it finds – from the bones, the teeth and the cells of every tissue. This borrowing is most unfortunate because the leakage of calcium phosphate accentuates weak bones. The mobilisation of magnesium is a source of chronic fatigue, headaches, loss of bone strength and hardening of the arteries; and the loss of calcium is not a stranger to the formation of insoluble salts which, on settling, form stones in places such as the kidney and gall bladder.

Many other factors are also susceptible to the

acidification of the body: overexertion of the liver, pancreas or kidneys leads to a poor breakdown of food; a hypometabolism due to a lack of vitamins, minerals and trace elements, stress and stones; a lack of oxygenation; or a poor pulmonary elimination.

By speeding up the rate of breathing and stimulating diuresis (urine production) through physical activity, particularly outside in the fresh air, we help to re-establish the metabolism of our lungs and kidneys, which are justifiably worn out by their hard work getting rid of acidic metabolites.

Malnutrition in the Overfed Developed World

Malnutrition is an obvious cause of illness. Contrary to what we might think, it's not only a problem for developing countries; albeit less visible, it is widespread in the wealthy, and often overfed and badly fed, Western world. Putting the situations of impoverished people for whom food is insufficient in both quality and quantity to one side, think about the slight figures of those who follow extreme restricted diets – the majority of fashionable diets unwittingly lead to nutritious deficiencies.

Most of the time, extra kilos mean surplus fats, and

a diet that is not tailored to an individual will not be a good solution, because most of the time it will make them lose muscular or bone mass, not to mention hasten associated health problems. Even a vegetarian diet can cause a nutritional imbalance; although a vegetarian diet isn't dangerous in itself, it can become so when the supply and the choice of vegetable proteins aren't properly balanced.

What Made the World so Fat?

The Western world is getting fatter before our very eyes. Recent figures are enough to worry us: in 2009, 32 per cent of over 18-year-olds in France – that's 14 million people – were overweight, and 14.5 per cent of them were classified as obese. And this 'guzzling' disease is growing at a rate of 6 per cent a year.

No one is spared, not children, teenagers or the elderly. A diet consisting of large quantities and poor-quality food is setting the scene for a large number of illnesses, increasing the risk of hormonal imbalances, cardiac incidents, diabetes and various types of cancer. These categories of illness are the cause of more than half of all deaths in developed countries.

The excess of fat is becoming a real scourge for all of us. Larger people are overburdened with visible fats, but the health of those who are smaller is also just as much in danger. Fortunately, illnesses caused by overeating can usually be prevented or treated by changing diet and lifestyle.

Anorexia: Inflicting Damage on the Body

This serious disease is down to major dietary imbalances. It has psychological origins and usually serious repercussions on the way someone eats. Nutritional deficiencies are obvious, as they are in cases of obesity, and anorexics, like obese people, can suffer from attacks of overeating. In the most severe cases, after each binge, the person will make themselves sick. In the morning their first reaction will be to dash to the bathroom scales which, they hope, will show fewer grams than the day before.

Of course, anorexia is accompanied by serious psychological issues. Most of the time, anorexics will not accept their shape, the curves of their bodies, or mostly they won't accept how others see them. It can also be a form of punishment young people inflict on their parents as a form of rebellion, impulsively eating cakes, sweets, ice creams, a whole assortment of food that they well know will make them gain weight, then stopping themselves from eating.

Often, young women who suffer from this sort of illness no longer have periods and cannot procreate: the lack of quality nutrients leads to a reduction in hormone patterns. It isn't easy to help them as they often can't help themselves. Treatment is long, sometimes uncertain, and there are frequent risks of relapses.

Problems for Men

Men are just as at risk from the consequences of a dangerous diet. This has consequences, notably on men's fertility, with a fall of around 40 per cent in testosterone levels. Through the centuries, the amount of physical exercise men do has fallen, a behavioural change that effects the self-production of certain hormones. A lot of industrially processed food contains female hormones, such as oestrogen, which, when consumed as part of an unhealthy diet, can undermine the wellbeing of men.

Between malnutrition, overeating and the cult of the ready-made meal, we privileged human beings in the Western world are no longer eating correctly. This is a shame, as the years that we're gaining, thanks to scientific progress and the variety of consumer products available, we are losing by devoting ourselves to the irrational appeal of eating unhealthy things.

Health Assurance

Family	Examples	Sources	Associated health effects
PROBIOTICS	Bacteria: Bifidobacterium bifidus Bifidobacterium infantis Lactobacillus acidophilus Lactobacillus brevis Lactobacillus casei Lactococcus lactis	Milk, dairy products	Helps the digestion of lactose Protects against infections (e.g. infectious diarrhoea, bacterial infections in the digestive urogenital system) Cuts the risk of chronic inflammatory illnesses Cuts the risk of food allergies
	Yeast (saccharomyces boulardii)	Yeast	Stimulates the immune system Improves intestinal motivity

Family	Examples	Sources	Associated health effects
DIETARY FIBRES	Oligosaccharides Polysaccharides Cellulose Starch Vegetable gum	Fruit, vegetables, cereals (roots of chicory, Jerusalem artichoke, wheat, onions, artichokes)	Improves the intestinal transit Stimulates colic fermentation Cuts juvenile cholesterolem Reduces post-prandial glycaemia and/or insulinemia Stimulates local immunities Affects satiation
VITAMINS	Vitamin C	Fruit and vegetables	Antioxidant properties: cuts the risk of cancer and cardiovascular diseases and cataracts

Family	Examples	Sources	Associated health effects
VITAMINS	Vitamin E	Nuts, cereals, vegetable oils, egg yolks, green vegetables	Antioxidant properties: cuts the risk of cancer and cardiovascular diseases and cataracts Help older people's immune systems
	Vitamin D	Dairy products, cod liver oil	Helps calcium fixation
	Vitamin B9 (folates)	Green vegetables, lentils, wheatgerm, liver, egg yolks	Reduces the risk of deformed embryos in pregnant women Reduces some risk factors for cardiovascular diseases

Family	Examples	Sources	Associated health effects
MINERALS	Selenium	Meat (beef, turkey, offal), fish (tuna, sardines, cod), whole cereals (rice, wheat), garlic, onion, cruciferous vegetables, mushrooms	Antioxidant properties: cuts the risk of cancer (particularly lung cancer) and cardiovascular diseases
	Zinc	Whole cereals, pulses, nuts, grains	Antioxidant properties: cuts the risk of cancer and cardiovascular diseases. Protective role in ageing

Family	Examples	Sources	Associated health effects
MINERALS	Magnesium	Dried fruit, chocolate, cereals	Prevents some complications with coronary thrombosis Reduces stress and fatigue
	Potassium	Fruit and berries, vegetables (especially potatoes), dairy products (except cheese) and nuts	Beneficial effects on hypertension

Family	Examples	Sources	Associated health effects
PHYTO-CHEMICAL MOLECULES	Polyphenols including flavonoids, isoflavones and anthocyanins	Soya, food containing soya	Antioxidant properties: cuts the risk of cancer, cardiovascular diseases, osteoporosis and inflammatory illnesses
	Phytosterols	Fruit and vegetables	Reduces cholesterol levels
	Sulphides/thiols	Cruciferous vegetables, onions, garlic, olives, leeks	Lowers the level of LDL cholesterol, protects the immune system

Family	Examples	Sources	Associated health effects
FAT CONTENT	Lecithin	Soya	
	Poly-unsaturated fatty acids (omega 3 and omega 6)	Fish	Reduces cardiovascular risks Reduces cholesterol levels
MILK-BASED PROTEINS AND PEPTIDES	Caseins (proteins a, fl and k) Lacto-serum proteins Growth hormones	Milk and Dairy Products	Reduction in the risk of thrombosis Anti-hypertensic effect on the arteries

Family	Examples	Sources	Associated health effects
MILK-BASED PROTEINS AND PEPTIDES			Regulates immunity Transports minerals Manages weight Antioxidant properties Anti-microbial activity Hypoglycemiant activity
SEA-BASED PROTEINS	Bioactive peptides	Fish, seaweed	Anti-hypertensive properties, immuno-stimulants, anti-cancerous, antioxidants

THE RISKS OF AN UNSUITABLE DIET

Family	Examples	Sources	Associated health effects
VEGETABLE PROTEINS	Soya proteins	Soya, food containing soya	Reduces the risk of heart attack Positive effects on bone health Beneficial effects on the kidney system Reduces the effects of the menopause Effects on hormone-dependent cancers
	Pea, corn proteins	Peas, corn	Allegations on protein content, improves intestinal transit

Source: Guide Nutri form 2005, 2006 and 2007, pages 101–120

CHAPTER SIX

PROTEINS AND DEPENDENCIES

As we've often mentioned proteins in previous chapters, notably warning against a diet that gives them too important a role, it's essential to better understand their relevance and their negative effects in the event of overconsumption.

Proteins enjoy a peculiar status, as if they are equipped with every virtue. For sure, they play an important role in the construction and repair of the body, because they make up the material structure of all living cells in tissues, organs, muscles, bones and skin. In fact, it's fair to say that, without them, we couldn't survive. But we must consume them carefully, both in quantity and quality.

Proteins and the Body

What is the point of the proteins that make up our bodies, and one fifth of our overall weight? The more we refine our knowledge of what's required for regeneration and recycling in the body, the more we realise the importance of proteins on a structural and functional level. To put it simply, they participate in the smooth running of all the cells – in the liver, bones, kidneys, heart, intestine, etc. – in which they're integrated, regulating their exchanges inside and out. Through this action, they play an essential role in the make-up of our organs. At the same time, they reign over our bodies by controlling our metabolic reactions. Each protein has a field of action and a destination organ. That's their fundamental interest.

They come from our food, and we find them in meat and fish, animal by-products like eggs, milk and cheese, vegetables, cereals, pulses and algaes. But, after they're absorbed, proteins must be subjected to a complex process of dismantling, then recomposition or digestion in order to become working proteins specific for the body. During this stage, the proteins are encoded with our DNA.

Note that not all sources of proteins are the same: it depends on their amino acid make-up. In effect, proteins are complex molecules, comprised of one or more (often more than 100) chains of amino acids linked by peptides. A peptide is the most simple example of a protein. Among all the amino acids that make up a protein, eight are deemed 'essential' – valine, leucine, isoleucine, threonine, methionine, lysine, phenylalanine and tryptophan. These are essential for our survival, but compulsorily provided through food, because, unlike other amino acids, the body can't digest them on its own.

A shortage in just one essential amino acid will have the same long-term effect as a total lack of proteins. Like the vowels in a word, essential amino acids are 'hinge' elements that cannot be ignored; without them nothing is possible. They rely on consonants, i.e. other amino acids, to make words, i.e. the peptides, and then make phrases, i.e. proteins. Proteins are therefore made up of various infinite phrases, all depending on the functions and organs they are designed for. And in each word we'll find the eight essential amino acids. To sum it up, amino acids make peptides, then peptides join together into proteins when they are all in a group. The opposite occurs at the moment of digestion, when food is broken down and amino acids are reproduced for different parts of the body.

Qualities and Characteristics

The main characteristic of proteins in the body comes from the fact that we lose them and consequently we must renew them. To be precise, the important protein capital encoded by DNA must be regenerated every 14 days. So our diet must contain enough of it in order to fulfil the perpetual and vital need of our organic functions.

Everyone is aware of the proteins' indispensable work in maintaining the muscular mass. To break this down, food sources with proteins have two other assets. Firstly, they make you feel full – all the nutrients, carbohydrates and lipids stay in the stomach for the longest and therefore take the longest to digest. Secondly, proteins require the body to put in a lot of effort in consuming them, so we therefore burn a few more calories during their transformation. To consume 100 calories of protein, for example, the body needs 25 calories to burn them and make them easy to absorb, while only 10 calories are required to burn a carbohydrate, and less than one for a lipid.

All food contains proteins, and there are a lot, all provided in different qualities and quantities. A greater understanding of them allows us to give priority to certain protein sources more than others. Remember that we need to find the essential eight amino acids in our food that are necessary for the body so it can make up its own proteins. During their growth, babies have a ninth amino acid called histidine that's uniquely contained in their food.

The eight amino acids aren't always present in each food at the same time. It's therefore important to diversify our protein sources in the same meal or during the course of a day. The benchmark protein source is eggs, and it's found mainly in the egg white. The value of all other protein sources is measured against the egg. All meat – beef, lamb, pork, veal and poultry (chicken, guinea fowl, turkey, duck) – and fish, and all their by-products, are excellent providers of 'complete' proteins, with varying quantities depending on the animal concerned.

We now have to distinguish between white and red meat. The latter poses a problem because it is high in calories, saturated fatty acids, cholesterol and iron (oxidising) and because of its acidifying effect. Too much red meat could bring about cardiovascular diseases and kidney deficiencies. In addition, cooking it at a high temperature (in a frying pan, under the grill or on a barbecue) leads to the production of toxic carbon compounds, which are proven to have carcinogenic properties, especially for the colon (see the Red Meat section in the ABC of Health at the back of this book).

The body finds it easier to absorb proteins from white meat (veal, poultry, rabbit). Fish, particularly salmon, sardines, tuna, anchovies and mackerel, is a great supply of unsaturated fatty acids (omega 3), which are excellent for health. Vegetable proteins – apart from soya, algaes and pulses – are not complete proteins; they lack three of the essential amino acids, notably lysine. However, we can easily get around this little shortcoming by bringing pulses and cereals together, for example, adding lentils or chick peas to whole rice (70 per cent cereal, 30 per cent pulses). This is a cuisine that vegetarians can perfectly master, but they need to consume it in significant quantities so that they have the sufficient quota of proteins, which can also stimulate a certain richness in slow-release carbohydrates.

Animal proteins are excluded from the dietary rules of our detoxification treatment, apart from those from fish, which is allowed twice a week. In common practice, we advise equal supplies of animal and vegetable proteins. At the end of this chapter, you'll find a table indicating the amount of proteins and lipids contained in each type of everyday food, the protein: calorie ratios (the higher this is, the more priority that product should be given in our diet). For your information: 100g of beef sirloin contains 28g of proteins and 6g of lipids; 100g of asparagus contains

2.4g of proteins and 0.2g of lipids. It helps to know these ingredients with regards to our daily requirements for proteins.

Our Daily Requirements

Our daily protein requirement remains a subject under discussion. The main problem resides in the turnover. To understand this properly, we must know that every day the body breaks down around 300g of protein, it recycles 80 per cent of it in order to form new proteins and only 20 per cent are completely eliminated or, to be more exact, they are transformed into urea and evacuated by the kidneys. It's therefore this 20 per cent of proteins that we must provide through our diet.

Up to this point, everyone is more or less the same. The difference comes when we look at the daily amount in grams. Usually, it's put wrongly at between 1 and 1.5 kilos of body weight. Here is where we don't agree at all. What is the weight that we must take into account? The total weight, as in the muscular, bone *and* fatty mass, or only the muscle and bone weight, otherwise known as the lean body mass? When we know that proteins only serve the muscles, bones and organs, we can quickly understand that it's lean body mass we must take into account rather than total weight.

As a consequence, we need to look again and lower the daily protein ratio. For instance, according to the commonly expressed hypothesis, a person who weighs 130kg, of which 45kg is fat, would need at least 130g of proteins a day. No. The person in question only needs 130 – 45 = 85g of proteins a day. If they have 130g, they will incur problems linked with the excesses we've examined. That said, it's extremely difficult to specify a precise daily supply, because it also depends on other factors: age, genetic profile, gender and physical activity.

We therefore recommend a supply of 45g a day for the average adult. New scientific publications extol the virtues of a supply not beyond 30g a day, even for high-level athletes. Again, they must fulfil their proper purpose, because to properly absorb all the essential amino acids they must all be present in a balanced amount in the intestine, and not only in the organs at the moment of their synthesis. The only way to achieve this is to vary and combine sources of protein in order to achieve the best absorption. When it comes to the best time for the absorption of food, remember that the ideal time is between 12 midday and 8pm (therefore lunchtime) when we should eat the most proteins, particularly as we age (especially beyond the cycle which starts at the age of 63). As a general rule, we advise people to begin their days in the following way: for a daily supply of 45g, have 7.5g in the morning and the evening, and 30g at midday.

Too Many Proteins

For all of us, there is a threshold beyond which ingested proteins are no longer used; they are then stored by the body after having been turned into sugars and fats. This protein residue causes numerous dysfunctions: a difficult digestive journey and an overproduction of toxic waste, often leading to constipation and colitis; excitability of the nervous and glandular systems; weakening of the renal and hepatic functions; acidification of the blood; excessive urea; and loss of calcium – particularly harmful for women and for those at risk of osteoporosis. Not to mention that these imbalances cause tiredness, requiring a supplement in the provision of water, vitamin B6 and potassium. That's why we're against high-protein diets. If they're followed for too long, or in repetition, they are guaranteed to cause health problems.

Too Few Proteins

When the body doesn't get its fix, it goes in search of proteins in our reserves, the muscles and the bones, causing cast-iron muscular risks and a fall in bone density, or even osteoporosis. Some shortages in essential amino acids can cause fatigue, loss of hair, broken nails, poor sight, fragile ligaments and immune deficiencies that lead to recurring infections. For children, any deficiency during their growth will always affect their constitution, because it can damage and diminish the production of the growth hormone. The same applies to those between the ages of 35 and 40: the loss of this hormone can have a negative effect on the quality of muscular tissues, and later, with the elderly, on bone quality.

Proteins and Age

As we have already seen, our ability to absorb and assimilate protein slows down as we age. The body finds it harder and harder to access its indispensable share of proteins because it becomes less efficient at transforming the proteins it's fed into proteins it can absorb. But should we therefore consume more? On this point we are categorical – no. But the more we age, the more important the quality and amount of ingested proteins becomes. By taking better control of the protein, we can also better control the age mechanism and the signs of deterioration in the body. This allows us to prevent problems linked to sarcopenia – the degenerative loss of muscular mass and the risk of tissue inflammation.

Remember again that, from the moment of digestion, proteins are subject to two opposing processes: their breakdown and then their synthesis or reconstruction. This dual action, which the body is less able to undertake effectively as it ages, causes the reduction of muscular force and mass, as well as the physical changes that follow. To clarify, the mechanisms that drive this loss in muscular mass are therefore of prime importance, particularly as the loss is also associated with an increase in fatty mass.

What should we do to ensure that our diet is as effective as possible in fending off ageing? On the one hand, the protein supply from food changes our metabolism. Our metabolism also fluctuates during the day because of the series of absorption periods, with a gain in proteins during eating, and post-absorption periods, when proteins are lost. A daily intake of proteins is therefore imperative in order to constantly maintain the level of proteins in the muscles and compensate for the lost proteins in the post-absorption period.

On the other hand, because the metabolism of older people no longer correctly breaks down the proteins consumed during meals, they must consume fewer of them in order to avoid the surplus that will putrefy and cause harmful waste. Remember that we don't go to bed one day and then wake up the next as an old person; the process is progressive and the reduction of the protein supply must be equally progressive.

Finally, given that the muscles develop a resistance to amino acids over time, we must become more selective and give priority to specific amino acids such as leucine, which increase the muscles' receptivity to amino acids.

However, the speed of absorption of these amino acids, and their beneficial effect on the metabolism, depends on the molecular form of the ingested protein. Prioritising proteins that are rich in small peptides is a nutritional strategy that's effective in preserving the good work of the body. At Merano, we favour lactoserum proteins (whey), which are rich and of good quality. This excellent product is taken in the form of a nutritional supplement, blended into drinks or soup.

We can see that regularly consuming proteins is important for the body, provided that an appropriate, controlled daily quality and amount is respected – but the real problem rests with adapting the ageing cycle.

Meat, Offal and Eggs

Per 100g	Protein:	Protein (g)	Calories	Carbohydrate (g)	Lipid (g)
Meat and offal					
BEEF					
Grilled steak	18.91%	28	148	0	4
Roast beef	18.91%	28	148	0	4
Heart	16.87%	27	160	0	6
Grilled sirloin	16.86%	28	166	0	6
Beefburger 5% MG	16.27%	21	129	0	5
Liver	15.86%	23	145	4	4
Tongue	7.96%	16	201	0.5	15
PORK					
Lean fillet	18.35%	29	158	0	5
Lean boiled ham	17.96%	30	167	0	5
Pork chop	6.06%	18	297	0	25
LAMB					
Leg	8.00%	18	225	0	17

115

Per 100g	Protein:	Protein (g)	Calories	Carbohydrate (g)	Lipid (g)
VEAL					
Escalope	20.52%	31	151	0	3
Rib	18.75%	21	112	0	3
Fillet	18.70%	29	155	0	4
Liver	15.33%	25	163	2	6
RABBIT					
All cuts	12.22%	22	180	0.5	10
POULTRY (skinned)					
Chicken (white meat)	19.32%	23	119	0	3
Guineafowl	15.33%	23	150	0	6
Turkey (lean)	11.11%	20	180	0.5	10
EGGS					
Egg white	22.44%	11	49	0.8	0.2
Egg	8.02%	13	162	0.5	12
Egg yolk	4.52%	16	354	0	32

Seafood and Fish

Per 100g	Protein:	Protein (g)	Calories	Carbohydrate (g)	Lipid (g)
SHELLFISH					
Scallops	21.69%	23	106	0	1
Prawn	21.42%	24	112	0	2
Lobster	20.83%	20	96	1	2
Squid	19.27%	16	83	2	1
Winkles	19.25%	26	135	5	1
Mussels	16.94%	20	118	3	3
Crab	17.13%	18.5	108	0.5	3.5
Oysters	13.23%	9	68	5	2
FISH					
Pike	23.40%	22	94	0	1
Monkfish	23.37%	18	77	0	1
Haddock	23.23%	23	99	0	1
Sole	23.07%	21	91	0	1
Black pollock	22.98%	20	87	0	1

Per 100g	Protein:	Protein (g)	Calories	Carbohydrate (g)	Lipid (g)
Whiting	22.82%	21	92	0	1
Cod	22.50%	18	80	0	1
Skate	22.47%	20	89	0	1
Dab	22.00%	16.5	75	0	1
Plaice	20.21%	19	94	0	2
Turbot	18.18%	16	88	0	2
Trout	17.96%	23	128	0	4
Sea bream	17.58%	16	91	0	3
Sea bass	15.54%	18.5	119	0	5
Carp	14.81%	20	135	0	6
Rock salmon	11.58%	17.5	151	0	9
Sardines	11.22%	22	196	0	12
Tuna	10.63%	25	235	0	15
Herring	10.32%	19	184	0	12
Mackerel	10.32%	19	184	0	12
Salmon	9.95%	20	201	7.5	13.5
Eel	4.82%	14	290	0	26

Vegetables

Per 100g	Protein:	Protein (g)	Calories	Carbohydrate (g)	Lipid (g)
Asparagus	9.60%	2.4	25	3.5	0.2
Spinach	9.20%	2.3	25	3	0.4
Beansprouts	8.29%	35	422	30	18
Cauliflower	8.28%	2.4	29	4.5	0.2
Watercress	8.10%	1.7	21	2.9	0.3
Mushrooms	7.86%	2.2	28	4.5	0.2
Brussels sprouts	7.82%	4.3	55	8	0.6
Lettuce	7.65%	1.3	17	2.6	0.2
Peas	7.22%	6.5	90	15	0.5
Artichoke	6.86%	2.4	35	6	0.2
Parsley	6.85%	3.7	54	7.5	1
Haricot beans	6.57%	2.3	35	6	0.2
Celery	6.17%	1.3	21	3.5	0.2
Cucumber	5.83%	0.7	12	2.2	0.1
Radish	5.24%	1.1	21	3.9	0.1

119

Per 100g	Protein:	Protein (g)	Calories	Carbohydrate (g)	Lipid (g)
Cabbage	5.19%	1.4	27	5	0.2
Salsify	4.93%	3.6	73	13.6	0.9
Leek	4.88%	2	41	7.5	0.3
Tomato	4.76%	1	21	3.7	0.3
Garlic	4.35%	6	138	28	0.2
Beetroot	3.66%	1.5	41	8.5	0.1
Onion	3.26%	1.4	43	9	0.2
Carrot	2.75%	1.1	40	8.5	0.2
Potato	2.35%	2	85	19	0.1

Fresh Fruit

Per 100g	Protein:	Protein(g)	Calories	Glucides(g)	Lipid(g)	Vitamin C	Vitamin C:
Redcurrant	2.39%	1.1	46	9.5	0.4	30	65%
Kiwi fruit	2.34%	1.1	47	10	0.6	80	170%
Raspberry	2.32%	1.0	43	8.5	0.5	30	69%
Orange	2.17%	1.0	46	10.0	0.2	50	108%
Lemon	2.12%	0.7	33	6.5	0.5	60	181%
Strawberry	1.89%	0.7	37	7.5	0.5	55	148%
Mandarin orange	1.86%	0.8	43	9.5	0.2	35	81%
Blackcurrant	1.85%	1.0	54	12.2	0.1	160	296%
Cherry	1.61%	1.1	68	15.0	0.4	12	17.6%
Apricot	1.60%	0.8	50	11.2	0.2	8	16%
Grapefruit	1.50%	0.6	40	9.0	0.2	40	100%
Plum	1.50%	0.8	53	11.0	0.2	5	9.4%
Banana	1.39%	1.3	93	21.2	0.4	8	8.6%
Papaya	1.36%	0.6	44	10.0	0.2	60	136%

Per 100g	Protein:	Protein(g)	Calories	Glucides(g)	Lipid(g)	Vitamin C	Vitamin C:
Guava	1.32%	0.7	53	11.0	0.6	250	470%
Peach	1.22%	0.6	49	11.5	0.1	8	16%
Grape	1.20%	0.9	75	16.0	0.7	5	66%
Nectarine	1.09%	0.7	64	15.0	0.1	24	37.5%
Pear	0.96%	0.5	52	14.0	0.4	5	9.6%
Pineapple	0.78%	0.4	51	11.9	0.2	26	50%
Avocado	0.73%	1.7	232	4.6	23.0	18	7.7%
Mango	0.63%	0.4	63	1.0	0.2	60	95%
Apple	0.52%	0.3	57	13.0	0.4	8	14%

Cereals and Dried Fruit

Per 100g	Protein:	Protein (g)	Calories	Carbohydrate (g)	Lipid (g)
Lentils	6.96%	23	330	56	1.5
Dried beans	6.23%	21	337	60	1.5
Pasta	6.11%	22	360	65	1.5
Cocoa powder	4.30%	21	488	38	28
Peanuts	3.99%	23	576	22	44
Porridge	3.64%	13.5	371	67	5.5
Almonds	3.49%	21	602	17	50
Bread	3.21%	8	249	52	1
Wheat flour	2.90%	10	345	74	1
Biscuits	2.70%	11.1	411	76	7
Hazelnuts	2.47%	14	566	15	50
Corn flakes	2.19%	8	365	82	0.5
Rice	2.14%	7.5	350	78	0.9
Dried apricots	1.75%	5	285	65	0.5
Dried figs	1.67%	4.3	257	62	1

Per 100g	Protein:	Protein (g)	Calories	Carbohydrate (g)	Lipid (g)
Coconut	1.13%	4.1	362	10	34
Prunes	0.78%	2.3	295	70	0.6
Dates	0.71%	2.2	315	75	0.6

Dairy Products

Per 100g	Protein:	Protein (g)	Calories	Carbohydrate (g)	Lipid (g)
MILK					
Skimmed milk	9.09%	3	33	0	5
Semi-skimmed milk	6.51%	2.8	43	4.5	1.5
Whole milk	5.22%	3.5	67	5	3.7
DAIRY PRODUCTS					
0% fat yoghurt	10.52%	4	38	4	0
10% fat cottage cheese	7.74%	8	60	3	1

PROTEINS AND DEPENDENCIES

Per 100g	Protein:	Protein (g)	Calories	Carbohydrate (g)	Lipid (g)
Fromage frais (40% fat)	5.24%	10	191	4	15
Yoghurt	4.08%	4	49	5	1
0% fat cottage cheese	1.75%	7	47	4	0
Crème fraîche	1.24%	3.5	282	4	28
Butter	0.09%	0.7	743	0.6	82
CHEESE					
Gruyère	7.74%	34	439	1.5	33
Munster	6.56%	21	320	5	24
Brie	6.27%	17	43	3.5	21
Goat's cheese	6.25%	20	320	15	20
Port-Salut	6.20%	22	350	4.5	27
Cantal	5.97%	23	385	5.8	30
Camembert	5.85%	17.5	299	1.8	24.7
Roquefort	5.84%	21.5	368	2	30.5

CHAPTER SEVEN

DOWN WITH TOXINS

The detox cure that I created more than 40 years ago has proven itself. Each day, I continue to perfect it in light of scientific progress and work especially on the ways to eliminate the surplus of toxins contained in the body. The ideal would be to feed ourselves so that food waste doesn't cause any more excess toxins. To achieve this, we must understand how they form and where they come from.

The Causes of Intoxination

In recent times, the word 'detox' has become a buzz word, often used by the media without them explaining exactly how the process works, as if it's merely a simple weight-loss plan, a seasonal clean-up or a baptismal-style purification. To a small extent, for the vast majority of us, toxins also come from the outside, from the surrounding pollution, the quality of air and water, from the rainy or the sunny weather, or from unsuitable cosmetic treatments.

Toxins are waste produced by the body, consisting of bacteria, dead cells and the residue of ingested and broken-down food. The abuse of some medicines (antibiotics and anti-depressants, among others) and the diverse harmful additives in industrial ready-made food also contribute to the accumulation of toxins, and to their impregnation in our vital organs via the nutritive (mesenchymal) fluid. Toxins are more than 80 per cent endogenous, i.e. produced by the body. They filter out into the principal emunctories: the intestine, kidneys, lungs, liver and skin, which naturally empty their waste through secretions, including stools, urine, gas, sweat and mucus.

For example, if the kidneys are overloaded with toxins, they can produce too much urea and uric acid, usually because of too much red meat. When the body can no longer carry out its eliminating work correctly, the surplus of toxins will clog up the cells – a process known as intoxination, which goes through various stages, from benign to more critical ones. It progressively opens the door to certain characteristic symptoms, and then a chain of events which can bring on more or less serious diseases in the long run.

The Saga of the Small Fish

In nature, we can find a good example to support our theory. To capture their prey, some small fish release an electric charge in order to paralyse them. However, if these predators live in a very polluted environment, they won't be able to act on their murderous instincts because they lack the energy to hunt. Result: they die of hunger.

It's a similar scenario when it comes to the body. The human body is a large emitter and a large producer of energy. Its emissions allow the liaison and transfer of data; cells, like organs, communicate between themselves on their own level, and the brain, with the help of the spinal cord, can send vital orders to the nervous system.

As long as the body dominates the amount of toxins that we produce, and it manages to eliminate them, then everything is OK. But the moment it becomes overloaded, toxins that it's constantly producing will invade the cells, weakening their polarity and therefore the ability to change and regenerate. We therefore feel tired and less energetic, and the balance between the production and the elimination of toxins is upset. This is what the concept of detox is based on: putting the body back into ideal conditions so it can do its proper work again, something the small fish cannot do.

As I broaden my professional experience at Merano, and thanks to the studies on homotoxicology (the science that studies the presence of toxins in the body), it's possible for us to define six legitimate stages of the penetration of toxins in the body, all with their own clearly defined origins and particular effects.

The Six Stages of the Intoxination Process

The extent to which the body is intoxinated forms the bedrock of an initial consultation between patient and doctor at the Academy of Biontology. It's an important indicator of our health status. When we feed ourselves in an unpredictable way, we play with fire. Getting this message across is one of the aims of this book: to understand and inform everyone how to prevent sinking our bodies into intoxination due to poor diet.

The first three stages of intoxination are reversible, and can be sorted out by rebalancing our diet; the final three, especially the last, may be more or less reversible on the cellular map.

The first stage is that of excretion, which mainly affects the workings of the stomach and the large intestine. At this stage, we mainly notice migraines and intestinal troubles, notably constipation. The second phase is that of oxidation, a reaction which principally affects the bladder and the small intestine, causing fevers and eventually bronchitis, tendinitis and arthritis, and there may also be changes in temperature and excessive and odorous sweating. The third stage is that of removal, which involves the hepato-biliary sphere, whose poor function has many side-effects: poor digestion, gas, heartburn, anaemia, demineralisation and a loss or gain in weight. The liver, the body's chief chemist, can also be subjected to worrying – but treatable – attacks: icterus (more commonly known as jaundice), hepatic colic, gallstones and even hepatitis. Watch out for this third stage: in effect, if the metabolism is very busy during this phase, it could lead straight through to phase six – the impregnation of toxins.

In these three initial stages, we believe that it's possible to act by closely analysing our diet, modifying our health and better regulating our meals, and respecting certain behavioural rules. With lots of discipline and a bit of good sense, we can achieve satisfying results pretty quickly.

With the three later stages of intoxination, however, we're entering into the domain of chronic illnesses and diseases of varying severity, which will greatly change our health and negatively impact our lives. The fourth phase is that of impregnation, which affects the lungs, spleen and pancreas. Alterations to the conjunctival tissue, a weaker immune system, lymphatism, asthma, allergies, chronic rheumatism and ulcers, among others, are the main characteristics of this stage, which we can often respond to with the more frequent use of drugs. This phase requires a long detoxification of around a year, and then a healthy diet followed to the letter.

The fifth stage is that of the degeneration of the vital organs: the heart and the kidneys. It goes without saying that any deterioration of these two organs can lead to serious consequences: various inflammations, risk of a heart attack, diabetes, arteriosclerosis, as well as neurological, motor and sexual problems. If we can't totally cure it, we can mitigate the damage by following a strict diet and regular detoxification treatments.

As we arrive at the sixth stage, that of neoformation, it's the liver that's affected the most, as well as the hormonal system. The whole body is now victim to a total degeneration of the cellular system, with the possibility of tumours forming. At this stage, the development of cancer can arise depending on the type of tumour.

Remember that the presence of toxins in our bodies is normal and, in fact, supported by our bodies – as long as their presence doesn't go beyond a certain limit. If it does, toxins can be a real danger to the body. They act as a destructive fuel that attacks and clogs up our tissues and our organs, turning the normal workings of the body upside down. So they must be eliminated.

On the Subject of Cancer

The more the environment (the body, cells, etc.) is clogged with toxins, the more its regeneration is affected. Depending on its terrain, if this worrying build-up of toxins isn't combated, it can slowly lead to a sort of anarchy and, in some cases, the development of cancer.

Recent therapeutic research has led us towards toxins that are naturally produced by certain plant, algae and reptile species that defend their natural environment. Using something bad to safeguard the good is useful, on the condition that the harmony between the two contrasting elements is always maintained. It's the same for the human body, as long as there's a correct balance between the production and elimination of toxins.

However, physiological modifications aren't always exclusively caused by 'material' damage, that is internal cellular pollution. The physiological impact of emotional shocks can also contribute to the development of some cancers, and treatment will involve therapy and surgery. On the other hand, regular detoxification before and after is necessary, if not vital. We must learn lessons and change our nutritional intake according to the risks of developing cancers.

Taking Toxins Seriously

Toxins aren't just a figment of our imagination, a mere personal suspicion or an anecdotal invention, but a proven scientific reality that is the subject of detailed studies and research.

When I first set out, I was greatly criticised for the validity of my methods. But, after almost four decades of practising the detoxification treatment, I am certain, and I have proof, that the proliferation of organic toxins that poison the body is definitely damage that could be avoided. It's vital that we get rid of them.

Researchers at the Institute of Genetics and Medicine in Naples have established a relationship between the intoxination process of cells and genetic diseases, particularly degenerative illnesses like Parkinson's and Alzheimer's. These revelations strengthen my argument: the inside of the cell's abilities to regenerate, reproduce and defend itself are harmed by toxic products that intrude upon it and have not been eliminated.

We've shown that this notion of intoxination is credible through tests which prove that, by detoxifying the body, the four most frequent ills –type 2 diabetes, hypertension, hypercholesterolemia and hypertriglycemia (which also happen to be most expensive to treat) – can be significantly reduced. This shows that, when we get our bodies working towards eliminating toxins, and they have the ability to do so, they will do so.

What can we do to help the body eliminate these toxins, and what can we do to ensure we don't overload our bodies with them? That's the object of our practical method, which we'll now spell out point by point.

The Detox Principle

Our benchmark course of treatment is an exclusive nutritional programme, combined with draining and energetic treatments, with the aim of revitalising the elimination of organic toxins.

It consists of a specific dietary procedure accompanied by herbal drinks that will give priority to eliminating toxins and minimising their absorption. This is not just a treatment of supplying the body with nutrients. Many different daily treatments personalised by a specialist team are given at the same time. Depending on the case, priority is given to certain areas of drainage, regeneration or elimination. This is why detoxification will always be something very individual, depending on the patient's age, genetic profile, current state of health, reactions and requirements. Depending on the problems that are to be faced, these different factors will demand attention on a case-by-case basis, involving modified diets and specific care during the course of treatment.

In fact, what we do is put the body in the optimal condition to eliminate the excess of toxins. After the age of 35, the body's ability to properly get rid of them diminishes because of the general slowing down of its metabolism, and of hormonal and digestive functions in particular. This diminishing process accelerates as each new seven-year cycle begins. Of course, the key stage of the treatment is a perfectly controlled diet. In detox, thanks to a specific dietary plan, we prioritise and accelerate elimination through natural channels: through the skin, intestine, lungs and kidneys. This activity is monitored by a medical team in order to assess the biological consequences on the body. Each day, the treatment includes sessions to balance the energy and the organs; manual body drainage combined with suction action; and capillotherapy, i.e. special baths with essential oils, wraps to encourage sweating and a toning shower to redynamise the vascular network.

The vast majority of toxins are circulated by blood capillaries. Therefore, these are what we need to stimulate during these different treatments so that they get rid of the toxins through their natural emunctories. We also look for lymphatic circulation using the same channels. The main objective of all the drainage treatments at each stage of our programme is the evacuation of toxins from the body.

What Results Can You Expect?

With problems of triglycerides or type 2 diabetes (non-hereditary), hypertension and cholesterol, the results are obvious, and all the symptoms reduce during the treatment. The secondary problems – notably fat around the abdomen caused by decomposition, fermentation and water retention – will improve after just the first few days of treatment. The detox effect is very quick when there aren't serious diseases to take into account.

Why is Medical Monitoring Necessary?

Our detox treatment is a serious plan that involves professional supervision, carried out by doctors, dieticians and trained medical staff. In addition, some diseases need to be medically monitored. It's also a way of assisting our patients, tailoring treatments for them and controlling their state of health throughout the course of treatment. Such an individually tailored approach means we sometimes encounter a blockage, particularly of the liver, which we can focus on in order to overcome it within three or four days.

Medical monitoring also allows dieticians to establish a specific dietary plan for the patient straight after the treatment – but this is not a diet *ad vitam Êternam* (for the rest of their life).

How Long Does the Treatment Last?

One week of treatment is ideal, once or twice a year. Seven days are enough to achieve a convincing result and to learn how to master – and stick to – your diet once you get home, with the help of our personalised advice. Some people with specific diseases can have the treatment for a maximum of two weeks. In just three or four days, on the other hand, we've only really done half our work.

Remember that you would never redecorate a house without cleaning it beforehand, and it's the same for the body.

Who is the Treatment Best For?

It works well for anyone who would like to remain in good health or who needs to rediscover a physiological balance and harmony, a new vitality or to change their diet (this could be for all sorts of reasons, including weight issues). For example, lots of high-level athletes come for a detox of their body before sustained physical efforts, and they are right to do so.

Stress, fatigue, a lack of oxygenation, inactivity, abuse of or dependence on medication like anti-depressants are all good indications that someone would benefit from receiving a treatment. After a detox treatment, we feel revived and we want to continue the efforts we've made.

Can Elimination of Internal Toxins Lead to Weight Loss?

Everything depends on the person and their physiology. Sometimes, there can be a spectacular weight loss, because the person loses retained, colloidal fluids which have gelled over time. During detoxification, they become fluids again and can leave the body. These fluids have a high toxin content and can create significant damage when it comes to cellular regeneration.

Losing weight usually requires more time than the week spent at the Academy of Biontology, all the more so because the origin and character of the excess weight needs to be examined first (see Chapter Four). Weight loss varies depending on individuals and their genetics, their hormonal changes, how active they are and, of course, the way in which weight was put on in the first place. We generally notice a loss of weight of between 2kg and 10kg, depending on the individual.

What are the Priorities of the Diet ?

Food, particularly meals with a controlled glycemic index, is fundamental to the outcome of our treatment. It is accompanied by plant-based drinks, water enriched with draining elements, vitamins, fibres and minerals that we prescribe to avoid deficiencies and optimise body drainage. Bread, coffee, alcohol, salt, sugar and refined products are forbidden, as is meat. It's a 40-year experiment in studying the role of nutrients, as well as a qualitative and quantitative strategy, that we put into practice.

Does it Have Any Anti-ageing Benefits?

Yes. The daily ability to regenerate cells is always involved in problems of ageing, which depend on the quality of the organic lipids. During the treatment, we definitely improve this regeneration, reducing the physical and physiological harm that occurs as we age.

Do You Also Have to Do Exercise?

Yes, physical exercise is always recommended. The amount and the duration are down to each individual, but in no case do we make it obligatory because the pace of the treatment is pretty tiring. Exercise is carried out in groups or individually and supervised by trainers. We also have some magnificent trails for a good hour's bracing walk in the fresh air.

Is Alcohol Prohibited?

The treatment does not include alcohol. Of course, when it comes to wine or other alcoholic drinks, it's the quantity that's the problem, not the strength. If we abuse alcohol, we are harming the chemical regulators of the liver and we're contributing to the degeneration of the fatty acids in the cerebral system. Everyone's very aware of the results: hepatitis or cirrhosis for some people, neurological or behavioural problems for others. A detox treatment has nothing in common with a withdrawal treatment. It is a natural, life-saving respite.

Can We See the Effects of the Detox?

We often forget, but the skin is the largest organ of the body and it plays a role in cleansing the body of impurities, just like other organs such as the liver and kidneys. This means we can often see the impact of a detox (and, equally, of a poor diet) just by observing changes in the skin. Acne, seborrhoea, sweating, redness, itching, eczema and psoriasis are the most common signs of an abundance of toxins in the body. The evacuation of toxins is usually carried out via the capillaries to the skin and then through sweat and sebum. More annoyingly, another way to rid the body of toxins is through serious inflammatory phenomena that occur in diseases such as herpes or shingles. When the skin can no longer get rid of toxins, it deposits them on the surface, which changes the appearance of our complexion.

During a detox treatment, we notice clients regain a clearer complexion, because of better oxygenation of the capillaries and the lymphatic system is unblocked, which enormously eases their elimination work. Detoxification slows down the ageing of the skin by favouring cell regeneration.

Can the Treatment Help You Stop Smoking?

There is no miracle in sight for smokers. We're all aware of the harmful effects of nicotine, tar and the thousands of other components of cigarettes and cigarette smoke on the lungs, the veins, the arteries and the heart. In truth, this list is much longer. The relevance of a detox treatment for this type of problem is very clear – it can be a trigger to stop smoking or, during the withdrawal period, help the body to partially get rid of accumulated tar. However, it takes many years (at least three or four) to ensure total elimination of the polluting tar from the bodies of people who have smoked for a long time.

ABC OF HEALTH

Rather than reluctantly list lots of recipes and diets, we'd prefer to share some sensible and wise rules, guidelines, advice and precautions on the use of food that's good and bad for your health, and on food and vitamin supplements, and their correct proportions, which have been proven in the fight against toxins. While some common habits and beliefs are overturned, others have been reinstated.

To be in good health, you need to be in harmony with yourself. Sometimes, illness isn't a coincidence, but a consequence of a bad habit. Illness occurs when this harmony is broken, and it can appear on either a physical or psychological level. The body is equipped with various means of recovery, and, as long as it's given enough time and the necessary nutrients for recovery, it will know what to do. If we give it the time and the means, the body will try to treat itself, totally naturally, when it recognises these imbalances.

This simple guide isn't trying to do anything else apart from help you to better understand the small things that can make a difference, and those things that we sincerely believe in. It is the fruit of all of our experience dedicated to the protection of good health, that all adults have a right to possess and preserve.

Antibiotics

There are some that you take as a medical prescription and some that are hidden in farmed meat as a result of being used to treat intensively reared livestock. Antibiotics represent considerable progress in treating infection and are the subject of continuous research. But abusing them, often pointlessly, only has bad effects: the body gets used to them and may build a resistance so they are less effective when genuinely required.

Remember also that antibiotic literally means 'anti-life': by killing different viruses, they also get rid of strong bacteria that is very useful for the proper functioning of the intestinal system. That which is damaged and thrown off balance must be restored to its proper state, in order to rebuild a solid intestinal flora. This is carried out by taking probiotics (starter cultures) during and after treating with antibiotics. Also be aware of excessive repeat prescriptions.

Assimilation

The more complex the bolus, the less effective the digestion. Not to mention the problems of the quantity of food being eaten. Indeed, there are mixtures of substances that contradict the rules of good assimilation. By mixing different food groups with different structures – for example, carbohydrates and animal protein – we are enormously complicating the body's work. It has to marshal different enzymes of different levels of acidity and alkalinity (more acidic for proteins; more alkaline for carbohydrates) to digest and assimilate such a mixture. This prolongs the assimilation time by creating a heavy feeling of bloatedness and sluggishness after meals. You can ease your body's task by following these suggested food associations:

Food Associations

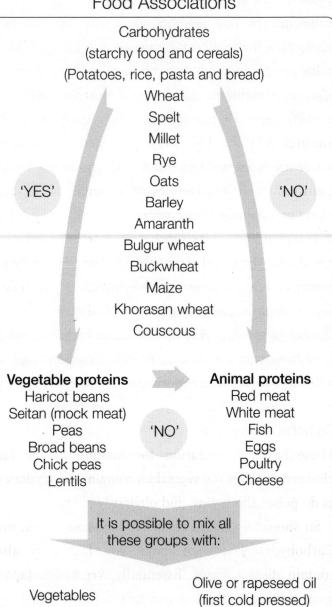

Carbohydrates
(starchy food and cereals)
(Potatoes, rice, pasta and bread)

Wheat
Spelt
Millet
Rye
Oats
Barley
Amaranth
Bulgur wheat
Buckwheat
Maize
Khorasan wheat
Couscous

'YES'

'NO'

Vegetable proteins
Haricot beans
Seitan (mock meat)
Peas
Broad beans
Chick peas
Lentils

Animal proteins
Red meat
White meat
Fish
Eggs
Poultry
Cheese

'NO'

It is possible to mix all
these groups with:

Vegetables

Olive or rapeseed oil
(first cold pressed)

Bathing

Balneotherapy is a method which has been proven, particularly in the effective drainage of macromolecules.

It's simply enough to completely immerse your body in a bath and take your bath at two different temperatures: 10 minutes at 36°C, then 10 more minutes at 39°C. This simple thermal variation of water allows a widening of blood capillaries, which contribute to the principles of elimination through blood and lymphatic circulation.

You could add three pinches of coarse sea salt or a few drops of natural essential oils. For a detoxifying effect, choose from essential oils such as lavender, thyme, cypress, cinnamon or citrus fruits.

After your bath, wrap up in a warm bathrobe, cover your head with a towel, then wait for 20 minutes in order to perspire and eliminate some more.

Carbohydrates

These have a reputation for making people fat. However, all fruit and vegetables contain carbohydrates, as do pulses and grains, and obviously potatoes.

So should we avoid them? A thousand times, no! Carbohydrates do not make you fat. They also contain dietary fibres. Essentially, vegetables (apart from potatoes), fruits, grains and pulses should form the basis of our diet. Again, it's all a question of quantity and quality.

When it comes to grains, it's imperative to favour the 'whole' versions and the same applies to all products made from wheat flour (bread, biscuits, cakes, tarts, pizza, pastries). They must always be in their whole form and never refined. Whole flour has a slow glycemic index (GI), whereas white flour has a much faster one and is neutralised by the insulin hormone, which always disposes of any surplus in the form of fats in fat cells.

Coffee

When coffee is roasted, the vegetable fats contained in its grains are oxidised during the roasting process. The roasting process draws out its delicious aromas, and, if it didn't have these bad dietary qualities, we could drink it to excess!

However, in very small quantities – two small cups of coffee a day, always served very strongly, followed by a glass of water – caffeine possesses some good qualities. It relieves headaches; it stimulates the brain; it's a light appetite suppressant; it lowers the risk of heart attacks linked to diabetes; it helps digestion if you don't have gastric problems; and accelerates the elimination because it's a light diuretic. But, let us repeat, too much coffee – like alcohol – is very bad for the health.

DIY Detox

Follow once a month for three days, or one day a week.

Purgative agent: one soup spoon of magnesium chloride mixed in a glass of water the night before starting the detox.

Breakfast:

2 seasonal fruits or fruit salad (200g)

Green or herbal tea

Lunch:

1 piece of seasonal fruit

Raw vegetables or mixed salad (a small bowl)

Basmati or brown rice, preferably organic (60/80g) and a small bowl of cooked vegetables

Vinaigrette of 1 soup spoon of olive or rapeseed oil and lemon juice and a pinch of fresh herbs

Afternoon:

1 piece of seasonal fruit

Supper:

1 small bowl of steamed vegetables with basmati or brown rice, preferably organic (60g)

To assist liver function and the bile ducts:

Herbal teas: bee balm, nettle, rosemary, dandelion

Vegetables: nettles (cooked leaves or in a salad),

dandelion, artichoke, rocket, chicory (endive) or other bitter vegetables

Herbs: rosemary, chervil, chives, sage

Infusion of bitter herbs + artichoke (you can find it in chemists and health food shops)

Spices: turmeric

Hepatic tea: dandelion, rosemary, artichoke, burdock and mint; drink one or two cups during the day

Evening Meals

It's important that evening meals are eaten early, if possible before 8pm, and they shouldn't be too heavy (see chronobiology in Chapter One) in order to reduce the possibility of becoming overfull. In this way, digestion will be quick, and the liver, having finished its daily digestive process of assimilation, will be able to properly devote itself to its overnight job of cleansing the body's toxins. Sleep quality will also be a lot better.

In the case of a late evening meal that is heavy and hearty and, moreover, accompanied by wine, this will hold back a large part of the liver's activity through difficult digestive activities, therefore compromising its nighttime cleansing process. Sleep will be heavier, with bad breath and a heavy tongue, and there will be slower secretion of the growth hormone.

Fasting

We all disagree with suggestions that fasting can be a therapy for your health, especially if it's a total fast that lasts for more than 10 days. It goes against all good sense, even if certain establishments have made it their speciality, because, depending on your metabolism, it makes you lose lots of mineral salts and trace elements. This in turn makes starting to eat again difficult, as the body is not in an optimal condition to process and absorb food. Much more serious among older people is the fact that fasting has the damaging effect of encouraging the body to eat itself, to the detriment of its muscular mass and bone density.

If in our centre in Merano we advise a period of fasting to certain people, it's always under medical control and never more than to facilitate the elimination of hepatic and kidney toxins. In all cases, it should never be carried out at home, on your own, as if it were a quick-fix, harmless treatment.

Fatty Acids

It is acknowledged that fatty acids allow the cell membrane, particularly the cerebral membrane, to acquire fluidity and permeability in order to maintain their capacity to function, to absorb the necessary nutrients for their regeneration and to eliminate toxins.

There are two categories of fatty acids. One is saturated fatty acids that come from animals (animal fats, cooked meats, butter and lard) and trans fatty acids (homogenised and oxygenised fatty acids), which have a large impact on reducing the quality of the cell membrane. We drastically need to limit their consumption. The second is unsaturated fatty acids, which beneficially contribute towards the correct balance in cellular exchange. These are, in particular, omega 3 and omega 6, contained in certain foods and which the body requires (for the right levels see the Nutritional Requirements table). The following foods contain these in good proportions:

Omega 3:

Animal source

Oily fish: herring, anchovies, sardines, salmon, tuna, swordfish, mackerel, trout

Vegetable source

Oils (first cold pressed): soya, sunflower, olive, flax, hemp, walnut oil

Pulses: lentils, soya beans, soya and pea seeds, haricot beans, red kidney beans

Flaxseeds (linseeds), marrow seeds, sunflower seeds

Omega 6:

Walnuts, cereals, wholemeal bread, rapeseed oil, eggs, poultry

Fruit

The time to eat fruit isn't at the end of a meal, because it slows down digestion; but at the beginning of a meal it can stimulate digestion. It's better to eat fruit in the morning because the body is in the elimination stage (from 4am to 12 midday), so before breakfast, or again during the afternoon in order to boost the blood sugar is ideal. You shouldn't eat more than two or three pieces of fruit per day, but should eat vegetables in addition to bring you up to the recommended 'Five a Day'.

Glutamate

This amino acid (glutamic acid) is naturally present in the brain and has a role as a neurotransmitter – it's essential for the memory. However, the food industry uses a distilled synthetic version that is unlike natural biological glutamate. Worse, it frequently uses it as a flavour enhancer, which creates an omnipresent poison in food. It's been proven that eating this product on a regular basis is dangerous for our health (side-effects include migraine, fluid retention, loss of hair among women), and it also means the tastebuds are incapable of identifying flavour.

Our tolerance threshold to synthetic glutamate is 5mg a day. We find it practically everywhere (soy sauce, biscuits, jams, ready meals). It's never

PURE HEALTH

mentioned by name on the labels on these foods, so memorise the following e-numbers: E620 to E627 and E631 to E637.

Gluten

When someone is intolerant to gluten, they need to cut out certain grains from their diet: wheat, barley, rye and oats. Wheat flour is present in the majority of industrially pre-prepared food (biscuits, flavoured creams, confectionery) where it's used as a binder.

We can be sensitive to gluten without being intolerant to it. This will mainly manifest itself in the swelling of the intestines when people eat too much pasta, bread, etc. Saturation follows, meaning the body can't get rid of waste properly. If this is the case for you, try to cut out gluten-rich food or reduce it over two weeks. If you notice that your stomach is feeling flatter after this period, you should limit your intake of food that contains gluten. Grains without gluten include rice, quinoa, corn, millet, buckwheat and amaranth.

GMOs (Genetically Modified Organisms)

In Europe, we're collapsing under the abundance of easily available food. We allow ourselves to throw away crops, and bins are full of out-of-date products that we haven't even started to eat. At the same time, over the past 50 years, we've had to feed an ever-increasing population.

If we set organic farming against intensive farming methods that misuse land and rely on pesticides to increase yield, we'd be right to choose organic. GMOs (genetically modified organisms) are allowed to be grown in certain countries on otherwise unfarmable land in order to feed all of their inhabitants and supply us with ingredients that frequently appear in our diets. It is dangerous to cultivate a dependency on GMOs.

We trust science when it's in the right hands, because we have every ability to put serious controls in place on products before they are released into the market. When it comes to grains, the finger has been pointed a lot at transgenic soya and corn because they are said to have harmful effects on the health. To be very honest, we have yet to notice the repercussions of this, though we're sure to have consumed them in meats from animals that were fed transgenic food. Disputes surrounding the problem are comprised of lobbying between ecologists and industry. At the Academy of Biontology, we feel that products coming from genetic manipulations shouldn't be put into the food chain and their impact on human and animal health be left as a surprise.

Hormones

A complementary hormone treatment is the best therapy to slow down ageing. It's a bath in the fountain of youth, for men as well as women.

As we age, the glands that secrete hormones get older and their production is less abundant. You can't help but notice their vital importance as you age, when their levels decline which can lead to heart problems, trouble with the memory, wrinkles, more frequent bone fractures, a fall in the immune and anti-infection systems, fatigue, a drop in libido, a tendency to get depressed, loss of muscle density, etc.

There isn't an anti-ageing hormone, though there is an anti-ageing hormonal polytherapy that brings together various hormones – gonadal (sexual), suprarenal, thyroid and others. These hormones – sometimes called 'life hormones' because they naturally appear in the body – also govern the proteins that we've seen are indispensable.

Hormonal therapy is still not accepted by the majority and isn't always well perceived by the medical profession. However, it has been proven in the treatment of diabetes with insulin, the menopause with estradiol and progesterone, as well as the male menopause with testosterone. Nevertheless, this therapy, which can bring certain risks depending on the person, requires an extremely specialist expert to assess what dosage to administer. It similarly requires thorough medical monitoring and assiduous adherence to the programme, so patients must be motivated.

Intolerance

Many illnesses which typically have an allergic origin with sudden manifestations, such as asthma, conjunctivitis, eczema, hives and allergic rhinitis, can be amplified by a food intolerance. Other illnesses can sometimes come from food intolerances that develop at different rates over time: neurosis, depression, certain forms of schizophrenia, headaches, epilepsy, hypertension, cardiac angina, obesity, gastroduodenal ulcers, ulcerative colitis, Crohn's disease, constipation, arthritis, dermatitis, acne and psoriasis. The full treatment of these conditions varies depending on the illness, but their extraordinary multiplicity shows that food intolerance can affect many functions of the human body. In effect, the toxins that form during this process target a particular organ, depending on the genetic predispositions of the individual, or the different disturbances they've been subjected to in their life.

Medicine these days certainly allows us to improve

the problem of food intolerance. It seems obvious to me that researching its origins should be more of a priority than therapy, because, once the responsible food is detected, all you have to do is cut it out from your diet, for life.

Kilocalories

At rest, some people burn 2,300 Kcal, others burn 1,300 Kcal, depending on the influence of genetics, hormones, physical activity and age. The lower this potential, the more you risk losing your shape, even if you exercise. As an indication: you consume 50g an hour at night and 100g during the day.

Lactose

This creates the same problem as gluten. When someone is intolerant to lactose, they must cut out milk from their diet, although they see much less of a problem with goat's or ewe's milk. Lots of people think – wrongly – that cutting out milk will lead to a lack of calcium. But there are other sources of calcium than just milk, such as vegetable-derived milks like rice and soya milk, plus oats, algaes and seafood products. Almond milk beats all the records when it comes to calcium concentration.

Lapses

Too much on your dinner plate means you have to take action the very next day. Beneficial regulation can be put into practice with a stock or a vegetable soup made from green cabbage, onions, leeks and carrots, a head of garlic (if you like it) and shitake mushrooms, which have a purgative effect. Green cabbage must be the main vegetable here, at around 50 per cent. Or you could settle for drinking a litre of stock during the day, then a few drops of lemon, hot or cold. Or, if the vegetables have been broken down, have the stock with them. You could also add 80g of wholegrain rice.

Magnesium

Stress and hyperactivity are big consumers of this nutrient, which is essential to the nervous system. Taking it as a supplement is a priority in cases of brain fatigue (under examination), failing memory, serious cramps and emotional shock. In our opinion, you should take it regularly in varying amounts – from 500 to 1,000mg a day depending on your sensitivity – preferably during a meal. The best quality is Magnesium Orotate.

Melatonin

This is a key manager of our hormonal system and constantly surveys the body's production and use of energy. Above all, it's a big regulator of our sleeping and waking cycles and our biological clock, controlling our daily cycles (24 hours), temperature, levels of cortisol (immune system) and the growth hormone and steroid hormones. Contrary to widespread belief, it doesn't make you sleep, but it can help you to regain a better sleep cycle.

On normal occasions, it's naturally produced by the pineal gland. As this ages, it weakens, producing less melatonin, which leads to a fall in the activity and efficiency of the immune system. After the age of 50, its production falls to almost 50 per cent of its peak, so it is beneficial to compensate for it through supplements.

At the Academy of Biontology, we consider melatonin a leading anti-ageing hormone, particularly because of its anti-radical and anti-stress properties. On the other hand, we have to find the right daily amount to take – usually between 1 and 9mg in the evening.

Metals (Mercury)

The poisoning of our bodies through metals is a major health concern. One of the most aggressive metals is mercury. In the past, it was particularly present in dental fillings, and today, this metal can be found in large fish, particularly tuna which, when eaten raw, can poison the body. Large fish contain it more than smaller ones; the older the fish, the more time it's had to accumulate metals. As it's essentially present in superficial fats, it's best to steam those products which may be tainted, so that the undesirable metals are destroyed. When we're affected by an excessive dose of mercury, we might have to undergo chelation therapy (the administration of chelating agents to remove heavy metals from the body).

Niacin (vitamin B3)

This is the vitamin that we should give priority to within the vitamin B group. It encourages a good supply of blood to the brain, thus decreasing the risk of mental illnesses such as depression and the risk of cardiovascular attacks. Above all, it increases sexual energy and protects toxins.

Its only inconvenience is in calculating and taking the correct amount, which is often recommended too low. The dosage should be fixed between 75 and 125mg a day, but it can cause hot flushes and some inconsequential redness. Niacine is naturally present in calves' liver, brewer's yeast, peanuts, salmon and tuna.

Nutritional Requirements

Recommended requirements for adults			
Substance	Abbreviation	Daily quantity/ allowance	Unit
Air	O_2		
Water	H_2O	1 to 1.2	g/kcal
Proteins, essential			
amino acids		1 to 1.5	g/kg body weight without fatty mass
Arginine (children)	ARG	circa 2.5	g
Histidine (children)	HIS	circa 0.6	g
Isoleucine	ISO	circa 1.8	g
Leucine	LEU	circa 2.4	g
Lysine	LYS	circa 1.7	g
Methionine	MET	circa 0.8	g
Phenylalanine	PHE	circa 1.5	g
Threonine	THR	circa 1.4	g
Tryptophan	TRY	circa 0.4	g
Tyrosine	TYR	circa 1.1	g
Valine	VAL	circa 2.1	g
Lipids		0.8 to 1.2	g/kg body weight without fatty mass

Recommended requirements for adults			
Substance	Abbreviation	Daily quantity/ allowance	Unit
Omega 9		Unknown	
Omega 6		circa 1.5	g
Omega 3		circa 0.5	g
Other unsaturated lipids			
Carbohydrates	100 to 150	g	
Minerals			
Sodium	Na	5 to 6	g
Chlorine	Cl	4 to 5	g
Potassium	K	2 to 4	g
Phosphorus	P	0.7 to 0.9	g
Sulphur	S	Unknown	g
Calcium	Ca	0.8 to 1,2	g
Magnesium	Mg	0 .3 to 0.4	g
Zinc	Zn	12 to 15	mg
Iron	Fe	10 to 15	mg
Manganese	Mn	circa 2	mg
Vanadium	Va	1.5 to 4	mg
Fluorine	F	1.5 to 3	mg
Copper	Cu	1 to 2	mg
Boron	B	150 to 200	mg
Iodine	J	75 to 250	Mcg
Molybdenum	Mo	50 to 200	mcg
Chromium	Cr	20 to 100	mcg
Selenium	Se	50 to 200	mcg
Vitamins			

Recommended requirements for adults			
Substance	Abbreviation	Daily quantity/ allowance	Unit
Retinol	A	1 to 3	mg
Beta-carotene	Provitamin A	2 to 6	mg
Thiamine	B1	1 to 1.5	mg
Riboflavin	B2	1.2 to 1.8	mg
Niacin	PP. B3	13 to 20	mg
Pyridoxine	B6	1.6 to 2	mg
Cobolamin	B12	2 to 3	mcg
Folic acid	M, B9	0.15 to 0.3	mg
Biotin	H	30 to 100	mcg
Pantothenic acid	B5	4 to 7	mg
Ascorbic acid	C	60 to 75	mg
Cholecalciferol	D	5 to 10	mcg
Tocopherol	E	8 to 12	mg
Quinone	K	60 to 80	mcg

Source: P. Forster

NB: Vitamins like vitamin C and B3 and minerals like magnesium need a higher daily intake.

Organic Produce

No reliable scientific study proves that products from organic farming have an impact on our health that's better than intensively farmed products. We're neither for or against – above all, it's a personal choice and a question of means.

Some vegetables resulting from organic cultivation actually develop toxic substances to defend themselves against outside attack. The best example is of the apple, which becomes covered with tiny black flecks that are particularly harmful to the body. In addition, as with intensive methods of cultivating and breeding, this expensive method of farming meets certain production problems. Can we still be sure that the product we buy is truly organic, because it can't be guaranteed that it was grown in complete isolation from chemical pesticides and growth hormones? But 'organic' has the virtue of attracting our attention to the varying qualities of products the food industry offers us, and it has gained a foothold for the methods of cultivation that are fairer on nature and therefore humans.

The ideal, when it's possible, would be to go for food that comes from farming that is guided, integrated and well managed, and which respects the seasons, output and price. On a global level, this is the best overall solution that would benefit the most people.

Physical Activity
If you already do this, good – continue to do it, but not to extremes. Too much exercise can lead to joint

problems and also a surplus of free radicals, which are factors of premature ageing that are both visible and invisible (within the body). For those of you who don't do it, it would be good to consider becoming physically active: one hour a day of fast walking, going up and down the stairs, playing golf or, for the more active, an hour of cycling or swimming, or exercise classes two or three times a week should be considered... it's not much to ask when you consider the benefits.

Indeed, there is more and more proof that regular exercise helps to slow down the loss of hormonal function. Production and retention of growth hormone, which produces lean tissue, diminishes with age. However, whether we're old or young, when we exercise it is secreted in the body. Furthermore, cortisol, one of the hormones that fights against stress, tends to stay too long in the blood of older people. Physical exercise helps to regulate it. Cortisol also balances insulin (the hormone that controls blood sugar levels) and, as we age, it allows the control of norepinephrine, a hormone that causes a loss of shape.

PRAL (Potential Renal Acid Load)
PRAL is a measuring scale of acidic power (per 100g of food), and it is scientifically determined through

the analysis of urine. A revolutionary nutritional concept, it possesses many advantages. Above all, it allows us to establish a precise measure of the acidifying power of food: the higher the PRAL, the more acidic it is. Below zero, the food is alkalising; above, acidifying. You should aim to balance both categories of food in order to obtain a final result that is as low in acid as possible.

FOOD	PRAL
MEAT	
Beef (lean)	+ 7.8
Tinned beef	+ 13.2
Turkey	+ 9.9
Calves' liver	+ 14.2
Rabbit (lean)	+ 19
Chicken	+ 8.7
Pork (lean)	+ 7.9
Dried sausage (e.g. salami)	+ 11.6
Sausage	+ 6.7
Veal (fillet)	+ 9
MILK, CHEESE, EGGS	
Butter	+ 0.5
Camembert	+ 14.6

FOOD	PRAL
Cheddar	+ 26.4
Hard cheese	+ 19.2
Soft cheese	+ 4.3
Milk (skimmed)	+ 0.7
Milk (whole/full fat)	+ 1.1
Milk (full fat pasteurised)	+ 0.7
Egg white	+ 1.1
Egg yolk	+ 23.4
Parmesan	+ 34.2
Whole fruit yoghurt	+ 1.2
Whole natural yoghurt	+ 1.5
CONFECTIONERY	
Chocolate (dark)	+ 0.4
Chocolate (milk)	+ 2.4
Fruit jam	− 1.5
Ice cream (vanilla)	+ 0.6
Ice cream (fruit)	− 0.6
FISH	
Whiting	+ 6.8
Prawns	+ 15.5
Turbot	+ 7.8

FOOD	PRAL
Herring	+ 7
Sardines in oil	+ 13.5
Salmon	+ 9.4
Sole	+ 7.4
Trout	+ 10.8
VEGETABLES	
Garlic	−1.7
Asparagus	−0.4
Asparagus	− 3.4
Broccoli	− 1.2
Carrot	− 4.9
Celery	− 5.2
Cucumber	− 0.8
Courgette	− 4.6
Mushroom	− 1.4
Cauliflower	− 4
Brussels Sprout	− 4.5
Spinach	− 14
Fennel	− 7.9
Green Beans	− 3.1
Soya Milk	− 0.8
Sea Lettuce	− 2.5

FOOD	PRAL
Lentils	+ 3.5
Onion	− 1.5
Peas	+ 1.2
Potato	− 4
Rocket	− 7.5
Lettuce	− 2.5
Soya	− 3.4
Tomato	− 3.1
FRUIT	
Apricot	− 4.8
Pineapple	− 2.7
Banana	− 5.5
Redcurrants	− 6.5
Lemon	− 2.6
Dried Fig	− 18.1
Kiwi Fruit	− 4.1
Unsweetened	
Orange Juice	− 2.9
Grapefruit	− 3.5
Apple	− 2.2
Pear	− 2.9
Grape	− 3.9

FOOD	PRAL
Currants	– 21
NUTS	
Almonds	+ 4.3
Peanuts	+ 8.3
Cocoa	– 0.4
Hazelnuts	– 2.8
Walnuts	+ 6.8
Pistachios	+ 8.5
CEREALS AND STARCHY FOODS	
Bread (average acidity)	+3.5
Flour (average acidity)	+7
Pastry (average acidity)	+6.7
Oats	+10.7
Corn flakes	+6
Flour	+8.2
Bread (rye)	+4
Bread (wholemeal)	+1.8
Bread (white)	+3.7
Pasta (wholemeal)	+7.3
Rice (white)	+4.6

FOOD	PRAL
Rice (brown)	+12.5
Rice (pre-cooked)	+1.7
Spaghetti	+6.5
FATS AND OILS	
Butter	+ 0.6
Olive Oil	0
Sunflower Oil	0
Margarine	–0.5
DRINKS	
Beer	+ 0.9
Brown Ale	– 0.1
Lemon juice	– 2.8
Grape Juice	– 1
Carrot Juice	– 4.8
Tomato Juice	– 2.8
Fruit Tea	– 0.3
Green Tea	– 0.3

Q10

This enzyme's fundamental role in cell regeneration and repair has recently been discovered, and rests on the unique condition that the daily dose is 100mg. Its effect has been notably demonstrated in problems with gingivitis. As a food supplement, it is an ideal precaution against effects of ageing.

Quinton Serum

This is, quite simply, seawater collected 5km from land at a depth of 800m. Quinton is the name of a French doctor who discovered the exceptional quality of seawater when it is protected from the sun's rays. Its composition is three times as rich in trace elements and minerals as human blood. Orally consuming one or two vials of Quinton Serum on an empty stomach each day is a unique blessing for regenerating the body and to achieve mineral balance. It is particularly beneficial for sports lovers, tired people, for those following a surgical operation or in the case of hypothyroidism.

Red Meat

The breakdown of animal proteins in the colon produces numerous metabolites (the intermediaries and products of metabolism), some of which are particularly toxic, such as carbolic acid, indole, ammonia and amines. With prolonged exposure to metabolites, the body can suffer carcinogenic effects.

So we must keep a close eye on our portions of red meat, without totally excluding them. In other words, we shouldn't have it in every meal or every day, just two or three times a week, and only in small quantities (150g).

Sea Salt

Everyone is aware of salt's main fault – it retains water in the tissues. Its role in the cause of hypertension is also far from minor. The snag is that there is salt that we can add for good use and salt that is hidden in various foods, including canned food, cured pork products, cheese and ready-made meals. So it is relatively easy to consume too much. However, in small quantities, salt is not without its benefits for the good reason that its composition of trace elements is very similar to that of human blood. We forbid industrial refined salt and other rocksalts in favour of natural sea salt. In contrast to sugar, it's easier to break our dependence on it. We should stop children from getting used to the taste of salt and not put salt on the table.

Seawater, Source of Life

Mineral composition (average mg/litre)	
Chloride	18,000
Sodium	11,000
Sulphate	2,600
Magnesium	1,300
Calcium	400
Potassium	350
Bromine	60
Nitrogen	10
Strontium	8
Oxygen	5
Boron	4

And in decreasing order		
Fluorine	Chromium	Tin
Argon	Antimony	Thallium
Lithium	Manganese	Thorium
Rubidium	Krypton	Hafnium
Phosphorus	Selenium	Helium
Iodine	Neon	Beryllium
Barium	Cadmium	Gold
Molybdenum	Tungsten	Thenium
Zinc	Cobalt	Lanthanum
Arsenic	Germanium	Neodymium
Uranium	Xenon	Tantalum
Vanadium	Silver	Yttrium
Aluminium	Gallium	Cerium
Copper	Mercury	Dysprosium
Iron	Lead	Erbium
Nickel	Zirconia	… and more
Titanium	Bismuth	

Sleep

Everyone is aware that good-quality sleep is synonymous with recuperation and regeneration. As we sleep, our bodies are far from being active. It's during the evening that the brain recharges itself with neurotransmitters that are essential for its proper functioning.

Unfortunately for those who sleep late, the best time to sleep is between 8pm and 4am: it's a fundamental biological rule. No one needs eight hours of sleep, so we can cheat by shifting it slightly later. It's good news for people who go to bed early who profit from regular cycles – first short (the REM phase), then lighter and longer – of daily rest. These one-and-a-half-hour cycles vary from one person to another – some need three or four, others five, in order to find their proper time of recuperative sleep.

All sleeping pills eliminate the sensitive phases – deep and light – reducing the quality of sleep and making it monotonous. A bedroom that's too warm, a poor positioning of the bed (the head should preferably be to the east) and synthetic curtains or carpets can also all have small effects on the quality of this crucial stage of the day. And, finally, exposure to lights or draughts can create harmful magnetic fields.

Vitamin C

This is an excellent vitamin and its overconsumption doesn't usually cause any inconvenience because it is water soluble – that's to say we don't stockpile it and it's easily eliminated via the urine, unlike other vitamins such as vitamins A and E, which are fat soluble and can be dangerous in large quantities as they accumulate fats.

However, we must watch out for the vitamin's quality – it should always be from a natural origin, such as that contained in acerola. Its beneficial effects are demonstrated in the healthy maintenance of the blood capillaries, bones and gums; a healthier absorption of iron; and the healing of fractures and urinary complaints. It also helps in the formation of collagen in connective tissues and in the fight against the harmful effects of smoking.

In short, it's a safe bet. The recommended daily amount is around 1g, all the while remembering the importance of hydration throughout the day. In our opinion, taking aspirin at the same time will slow down its absorption. Symptoms of a lack of vitamin C include weakness in the muscles; fatigue; hypotension; swelling of the gums; and digestive difficulties. Find it in good proportions in certain fruit (kiwi fruit, citrus fruits, berries and papaya), in parsley and in cooked cabbage.

Water
This is the major element in life. It's also the main conductor of energy which, along with the blood, allows the transportation of nutrients and helps the elimination of organic waste.

Our average requirement of this special fluid is around 1.5 litres a day, including other drinks (tea, fruit or vegetable juice, etc.). The sensation of thirst diminishes with age – a problem that's not without its risks, especially on very hot days, and if the person concerned is on diuretics. So you have to be careful. We strongly advise everyone to enrich their daily water intake with either cider vinegar (1 soup spoon for every 1.5 litres of water) in order to help drainage and hepatic channels, or the juice of half a lemon to stabilise the blood pH level.

Z

Zero faults in our diet, that's what we should strive for every day. Eat regular meals, keep an eye on how much you eat, prioritise certain food and get rid of others, respect the right time for sleeping, watch your weight (fat), stop snacking – especially on food containing fast-releasing sugars – keep your brain active, get some fresh air, walk and be in control of your emotions: these are the fundamental rules for a good, healthy life.